ACETABULARIA AND CELL BIOLOGY

Acetabularia and Cell Biology

S. PUISEUX-DAO

Professor of Cell Biology
University of Paris

Translated by

Dr. P. Malpoix-Higgins,
Université Libre de Bruxelles

SPRINGER—VERLAG NEW YORK INC.

LOGOS PRESS LIMITED

Sole Distributor for the United States of America,
its territories and possessions,
the Philippine Republic and Canada

SPRINGER—VERLAG NEW YORK INC.

Library of Congress Catalog Number 77-80927

Title Number 8-8002⬧

© S. Puiseux-Dao, 1970

Printed in Great Britain by
The Garden City Press Limited
Letchworth, Hertfordshire

CONTENTS

PREFACE

During the First International Symposium on *Acetabularia*, held last June in Brussels and Mol, one question emerged repeatedly, and was hotly disputed: Is *Acetabularia* a cell or an organism? One of the beauties of *Acetabularia* is that you can have it both ways: it has all the attributes of a giant plant cell (nucleus, chloroplasts, mitochondria, ribosomes, etc.) and, on the other hand, it has a cell cycle during which gametes and zygotes are formed. During this reproductive period, the alga is multinucleate and truly behaves as a unicellular, multinucleate organism; during the preceding period of growth, it has a single nucleus and it behaves very much like a cell.

But it is a very queer cell indeed: it is truly gigantic, several centimeters long. In its big nucleus, the nucleolus is ribbon shaped, unusually large and contains a high quantity of ribonucleic acid (RNA). Still much stranger is the ability of the uninucleate alga to undergo morphogenesis and to produce a lovely 'cap' or 'umbrella' which will serve for its gametic reproduction.

However, *Acetabularia* would not be the subject of a book without the pioneer work of *Hämmerling* on its *regeneration*: his experimental curiosity led him to cut off the stalk of algae prior to cap formation; he discovered that the anucleate fragments are not only able to survive for many weeks, but can even produce normal caps. Since the cap is typically species specific, it is clear that its production and its shape are genetically controlled. The paradox is that a genetically determined character is expressed although all the genes have been removed by surgical excision of the nucleus. To explain this regeneration in the absence of the nucleus, Hämmerling postulated the production of '*morphogenetic substances*' by the nucleus; they would be stored in the cytoplasm, where they would retain for a long time what we would now call the genetic information. Further experiments by Hämmerling, in which the algae were cut into three or more pieces, demonstrated that the morphogenetic substances are distributed along an apicobasal decreasing gradient (although the nucleus lies in the rhizoid, at the basal end of the alga). More elaborate experiments of inter-specific grafts, in which the nucleate half of one species was fused together with the anucleate fragment of another species, gave conclusive proof that the 'morphogenetic substances' are really produced by the nucleus and that they are species specific (Hämmerling, 1934).

When my Colleague Professor H. Chantrenne and myself became interested in the biochemistry of *Acetabularia* in 1955, we did not realise that we were following in the footsteps of Alice in Wonderland: we first looked, without much hope, for a net *protein synthesis* in the anucleate fragments and found it. In fact, the protein content of these fragments more than doubles within one month. Still more surprising was the fact that there are several functional enzymes among the synthesised proteins. We knew since Beadle's famous slogan 'one gene, one enzyme' that the synthesis of these enzymes is genetically controlled; how is such a synthesis of specific proteins possible when there are no genes in the synthesising system?

This paradox led me, in 1960, to the suggestion that the 'morphogenetic substances' might be molecules of RNA, which would be produced in the nucleus, transferred into the cytoplasm and stored, in a very stable form, at the apex of the stalk where they would retain their genetic information for a very long time. This suggestion was made a few months before the messenger RNA (m-RNA) theory came to light; the idea was essentially the same, except that it was believed, at that time, that m-RNAs always have a short lifetime. We now know that this is not necessarily so; it is therefore now generally assumed that *Hämmerling's morphogenetic substances are stable m-RNAs.*

What happens to the *nucleic acids*, RNA and DNA, in the anucleate fragments of *Acetabularia*? After some controversy, there is now perfect agreement between the groups working in Wilhelmshaven and in Brussels about the answer to this question: there is a marked RNA synthesis in the anucleate halves, and the same species of RNA are produced in the two kinds of fragments. Still more surprising is the fact that the anucleate fragments not only contain DNA, but can replicate it.

The solution of this new paradox came when it was found (Brachet and Baltus; Gibor and Izawa) that the chloroplasts of *Acetabularia* contain DNA and that these chloroplasts can increase in number in the absence of the nucleus (Shephard). A large amount of work, which will be described in the book, has been devoted to the question of the autonomy of the chloroplasts in *Acetabularia*. The answer is that, thanks to their own DNA, the chloroplasts do not depend entirely upon the nucleus, but that they 'do better' in nucleate than in anucleate halves: in other words, chloroplasts behave more like symbionts than parasites. This conclusion has been reinforced by the fact that, according to Janowski and Bonotto, polysomes can be formed in the cytoplasm of *anucleate* halves: in these polysomes, the ribosomes are probably of nuclear (nucleolar) origin, while the m-RNAs apparently come from the chloroplasts.

Coming back to the equation 'morphogenetic substances = stable m-RNA', it should be pointed out that it remains an attractive hypothesis, which agrees with our present thinking in molecular biology, but which is supported by indirect evidence only: it agrees with the experimental results obtained when nucleate and anucleate fragments of the algae are treated with actinomycin (an inhibitor of DNA-primed RNA synthesis) and with the fact, discovered by Farber and by Janowski, that certain RNA species remain undegraded for more than three months in the algae. But direct proof will not be obtained until the alleged m-RNAs (it is likely that the nucleus produces many different species of m-RNAs, in view of the structural and chemical complexity of the caps) have been isolated and proven, by micro-injection experiments, to be responsible for morphogenesis in the absence of the nucleus.

There is still a long way to go before we reach that goal and we need a milestone on the road: it is provided by the present book which comes at the right time. Nobody could have been a better author than Professor S. Puiseux-Dao, who has an excellent background in botany (especially in algology), has worked both in Wilhelmshaven and in Brussels, and has brought important personal contributions to the subject (her recent work on the 'plastidial units' is of very great importance for the understanding of the interactions between the nucleus and the chloroplasts). The book is clearly written, well thought out and really up to date. The extensive and very complete bibliography will prove extremely useful to all those interested in the subject. Despite the many problems which have faced the author (in May 1968 in Paris, the creation of a department in the new Faculty in Montrouge which is still in its experimental stage), she has beautifully succeeded in her work. Recognition to an appreciable extent in the success of the book should go to the translator, Dr. Pamela Malpoix, who shares a perfect command of both the English and the French languages and a good personal knowledge of the subject.

It is to be hoped that, after reading the book, many research workers will be enticed to participate in the unravelling of the secrets of this mysterious and fascinating organism, *Acetabularia*.

Brussels   J. BR ACHET
December 1969

The author would like to acknowledge the skilful assistance of Anne-Marie Blondel with the drawings.

1

Introduction

The *Acetabularia*, Chlorophyceae, belong to a strange but homogeneous order of algae, the Dasycladales, fossil examples of which date from early Silurian, many of these algae being calcified. They occur in calm, fairly warm seas, generally anchored to pebbles or sea-shells on sandy sea-beds in shallow water, at depths varying from a few inches to several feet.

The morphology and life history of the best known species, *Acetabularia mediterranea*,* was described in 1877 by de Bary and Strasburger. The reproductive organ or cap is formed at the apex of the axial siphon; the rounded cysts which develop in it are released after a variable period of rest as biflagellate zoids. The latter are capable of producing a plant identical to the original parent, either by direct germination or after fertilisation (de Bary and Strasburger, 1877). The life cycles of all *Acetabularia* so far studied seem to be identical.

Hämmerling (1932) was the first to achieve successful cultures of *Acetabularia* on a fairly large scale (1931). His culture techniques are based on those elaborated by algologists working with marine biological material. Although fairly efficient, the cultures have two major disadvantages: the use of enriched sea water or 'Erdschreiber', the composition of which was not sufficiently well defined, and lack of sterility. Indeed, such cultures are always contaminated by Bacteria and sometimes by Protista. Infection can be avoided during periods of limited duration, but cannot be permanently eliminated, because of the slow rate of growth which characterises this alga.

The discovery that *Acetabularia* is in fact a single giant uninucleate cell growing at the apex and capable of morphogenesis was also due to Hämmerling (1932); in some species this single uninucleate cell reaches a length of several tens of millimetres. While this feature seems to be characteristic of all

---

* The species is now known as *A. acetabulum*.

Acetabularia, it is still an open question whether the single nucleus is diploid or polyploid. The alga remains uninucleate until the reproductive cap is completely formed; the single nucleus then breaks up into numerous daughter nuclei which are carried by cytoplasmic streaming to the reproductive organ at the tip of the stalk. The cysts are formed there by the enclosure of each new nucleus.

The giant uninucleate cells of *Acetabularia* have frequently been used as particularly suitable biological material for the study of nucleocytoplasmic relationships. Morphogenetic studies of nucleate and anucleate fragments enabled Hämmerling (1932) to demonstrate the capacity of the cytoplasm to survive and retain remarkable morphogenetic potentiality, including the power to produce an externally normal reproductive cap, after removal of, and in the absence of, the nucleus. His beautiful and now famous, intra- and interspecific graft experiments confirmed this finding (1943b) and led to the conclusion that long-lived morphogenetic substances of nuclear origin, with species specificity, are stocked in the cytoplasm.

These experiments could not fail to awaken the interest of another worker, Brachet (1941), who had already proposed an interesting, but then revolutionary hypothesis, suggesting the existence of a relationship between the nucleic acids in the nucleus and the cellular synthesis of proteins. In spite of the difficulty encountered in obtaining sufficiently large quantities of algae, biochemical experiments were begun on nucleate and anucleate fragments. Completed by various analytical techniques, especially enzymatic tests in Brachet's Belgian laboratory, then in Hämmerling's German one, this work brought evidence of a special role for the nucleus in the synthesis not only of proteins, but also of nucleic acids. The significance of these results became even more evident when later work on Bacteria, including *Escherischia coli*, accurately established the nature of the genetic code in chemical terms, and furnished a logical explanation for the relationship between DNA, RNAs and protein.

It was nevertheless quite obvious that nucleocytoplasmic relations in Eucaryotes like *Acetabularia* must be much more complex than in Bacteria. In order to localise the sites of synthesis of the different types of RNAs and to try to discover the meaning of nucleocytoplasmic exchange, autoradiographic methods were perfected in Brachet's laboratory (1957). Pulse and chase experiments effectively revealed that part of the cytoplasmic RNA came from the nucleus, being accompanied in its migration by basic proteins and proteins rich in sulphur groups. The fact that these molecules of RNA and protein, associated together to a variable extent, were localised in the cytoplasm and particularly concentrated at the apex of the stalk, suggested that they could be identified with the morphogenetic substances of Hämmerling.

Further morphological, biochemical and autoradiographical studies were performed on algae in which the fundamental metabolic pathways affecting the circuit DNA-RNAs-proteins was disturbed at some precise step by specific inhibitors like ribonuclease, actinomycin and puromycin. The results so obtained are in no way at variance with the idea that the morphogenetic substances are homologous with long-lived messenger RNAs of nuclear origin, protected and stabilised, perhaps, by their association with basic proteins. Naturally, on further examination, the situation was found to be much more complex. First, it became clear from research carried out on amphibian embryos and other animal cells that the precursors of hyaloplasmic ribosomes are probably synthesised in the nucleolus. Among the RNA-protein complexes leaving the nucleus of *Acetabularia*, it therefore became necessary to distinguish those which correspond to ribosomes, and those which correspond to actual nuclear 'messages'. Moreover, the discovery that cytoplasmic organelles are highly autonomous made evident the vital role they must play in nucleocytoplasmic relations; although the interpretation of a certain number of experimental results was facilitated by this finding, the overall picture became correspondingly more confused.

In fact, mitochondria and chloroplasts have their own DNA, under the control of which they are able to synthesise proteins, as has been shown by experiments involving the incorporation into these organelles (isolated from various biological materials, including *Acetabularia* (Brachet and Goffeau, 1964)) of radioactive precursors of RNAs and proteins, in the presence or absence of actinomycin. Rather small plastids are particularly abundant in the not very dense cytoplasm of these algae. Their synthetic capacity seems to be one of the main factors ensuring the survival of anucleate fragments. They are composed of fairly well delimited units, the multiplication of which, like the photosynthetic activity of the alga, follows a temporal rhythm. The diurnal-nocturnal periodicity which is typical of some plastidal functions is endogenous and subject to nuclear control. Analysis of this nuclear control now constitutes one of the best ways of investigating the relations between cytoplasmic organelles containing this so-called 'satellite' DNA* and nuclear DNA.

An understanding of control mechanisms, particularly those directing the synthesis of proteins in the cytoplasm, is at present a basic preoccupation of laboratories working on *Acetabularia*. Indeed, the functional autonomy of the plastids may well contribute to the survival of anucleate cytoplasm by maintaining a source of carbon chains and energy, but it is unlikely to preserve the genetic messages responsible for specific morphogenesis and ensure their translation. Sequential derepression of new functions, parallel to the cessation of earlier metabolic pathways, occurs during the lifetime of the alga; the two main subdivisions of this process are first the growth period, during which a particular type of cell wall is elaborated, and second, the reproductive phase during which another type of cell wall with a different chemical composition is formed, characteristic of the cap. The regulation of these two main stages seems to be a purely cytoplasmic phenomenon, and its understanding will certainly throw light upon one of the fundamental problems of cell differentiation.

It has been possible to approach a number of essential biological problems through the study of *Acetabularia*. Its well defined morphology has made it possible to demonstrate the extreme limit of cytoplasmic autonomy and to show its dependence upon substances of nuclear origin containing RNA. Autoradiography has brought evidence of the fact that these RNAs are associated with proteins and are very precisely located in the cell. Although *Acetabularia* lends itself very readily to morphological and cytological observation, it is not a very

---

* The term 'satellite' derives from the biochemical techniques which first enabled such DNA, sometimes different in buoyant density from nuclear DNA, to be separated from it by ultracentrifugation in CsCl gradients.

• •

favourable material for biochemical study, owing to the difficulty of obtaining large supplies. Moreover, like most algae, its high water content makes biochemical assays more difficult, as do bacterial contaminants which are frequent. It has nevertheless been possible to achieve such assays and to interpret, by comparison, the former kind of experiment in a satisfactory way. The above mentioned difficulties, as well as the prolonged life cycle of the algae (four to nine months for one single generation), which renders genetic studies impossible, have caused a good deal of pessimism in scientific circles. Nevertheless, *Acetabularia* remains a most suitable object for the study of the relations between the nucleus and the plastids, and of the interdependence between the cytoplasm and the nucleus: if the reproductive cap is cut during the process of maturation, nuclear division is prevented. Moreover, few biological materials are so useful for the study of nuclear and messenger RNAs, of their fate in the cytoplasm, and of the way in which normal cell differentiation is ensured by their ordered translation, even in the absence of the nucleus.

The biology of *Acetabularia*

A. MORPHOLOGY AND MORPHOGENESIS IN *ACETABULARIA*

1. Morphology and morphogenesis in Acetabularia mediterranea

The best known species of *Acetabularia* is *Acetabularia mediterranea*. These algae can be harvested along the mediterranean coast and in brackish lakes along the littoral. The size and shape of their calcified, discoid, umbrella-like reproductive cap, measuring about 1 cm in diameter, makes them easily recognisable. Each reproductive cap terminates a thin cylindrical stalk encrusted with calcium carbonate, and reaching a height of 3 to 6 cm, whereas the basal rhizoid is about 1 mm in diameter. The stalk is firmly anchored to shells, pebbles or rocks by several rhizoids. Each total unit composed of: rhizoids, cylindrical stalk and cap, constitutes the adult alga (Fig. 1). The young plants do not possess caps, but only a few ramified hairs; they germinate from zygotes and sometimes zoospores.

In culture, under favourable conditions (de Bary and Strasburger, 1877; Hämmerling, 1931; Puiseux-Dao, 1962), the youngest stages resemble bright or dark green balls which are more or less spherical in shape and 2 to 10 μ in diameter. Many of the little plants grow rapidly and acquire cylindrical shape within a few days, whereas others may remain static in development for much longer periods and may only start to grow after several months' delay. Right from the beginning, growth clearly occurs preferentially at one, usually light and pointed pole of the tiny cylinder. The other extremity of the alga changes only slowly in aspect: after a few weeks it forms irregular branches, the rhizoids, the membranous coat of which gradually increases in thickness (Fig. 1). The rate of growth accelerates progressively: within three to five months the stalk

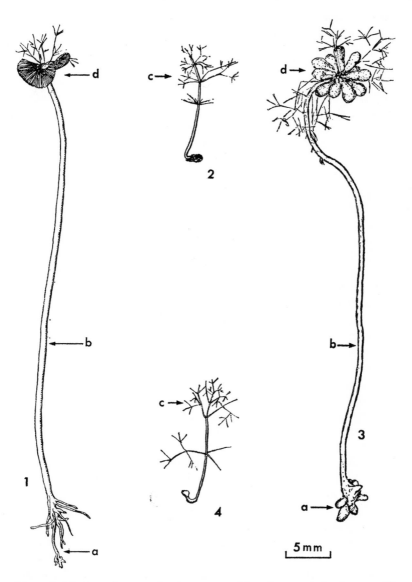

Figure 1. (1) *A. mediterranea* in the process of forming a reproductive cap. (2) Young plant of *A. mediterranea*. (3) Adult *A. peniculus*. (4) Young plant of *A. peniculus*: (a) rhizoids; (b) axial stalk; (c) sterile whorls; (d) reproductive cap (culture algae).

has increased in length from 100 μ to 4 cm or more, while the diameter has risen from 50 to 500 μ, the apex always remaining finer than the rest of the stalk.

As soon as the alga measures a few millimetres, whorls of eight to ten branches of hair-like members make their appearance at more or less regular intervals; at first widely spaced, they later become closer together. They emerge at the rounded or flattened apex as a circle of swellings which lengthen, become cylindrical, then basally constricted at their point of junction with the stalk. When the first hairs have almost reached their maximum length, which is about a millimetre, several new rudiments appear in their distal region and grow into fine threads resembling, in miniature, those from which they have been formed; a basal constriction appears in the same manner. These are the 'second order' branches, which will similarly give rise to two or three further dichotomies. This process may in fact be repeated until the whorls bear fifth or sixth order branches. Little by little, the communicating pores are obstructed by colourless substances and the branches finally drop off, beginning with the most distal hairs, each whorl leaving a ring-shaped scar on the stalk (Fig. 2). At first the hairs seem to prolong the stalk, but the growth of the apex recommences as soon as second order branches appear on the whorl. The elongation and thickening of the apex alters the arrangement of the initially formed members, which spread out to such an extent that they become almost perpendicular to the stalk. The repetition of this phenomenon on a minor scale at each branching results in widely deployed whorls. The apical cell wall thickens to such an extent that it causes the hairs to disappear at their point of constriction, leaving a hollow scar.

When, after six months culture or more, the algae attain an average size of 4 to 6 cm they form two to four consecutive, tightly juxtaposed, sometimes overlapping whorls; cap initiation begins by the flattening of the apex, which becomes externally striated to form the superior corona beneath which a series of tightly packed globular protuberances will form the inferior corona and the reproductive chambers (Solms-Laubach, 1895; Howe, 1901). Like the hairs, these outgrowths become partially separated from the axial stalk by annular obturation; their thickened bases persist at the top of the stalk to form the

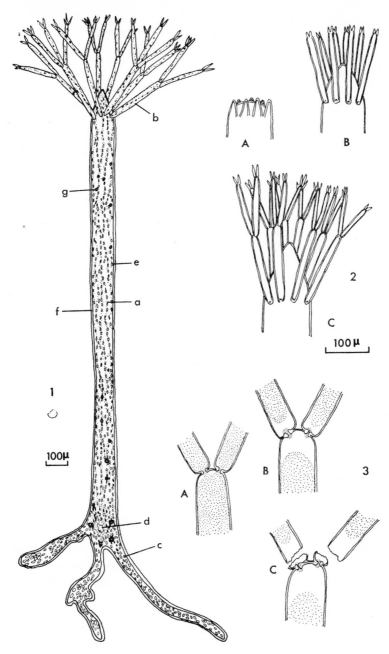

Figure 2. (1) Young plant of *A. mediterranea*. (a) axial stalk; (b) sterile whorls; (c) rhizoids; (d) nucleus; (e) plastid; (f) membrane; (g) lipid drop. (2) Formation of sterile whorls. (3) Deciduation of branching hairs. (After Puiseux-Dao, 1962.)

'vestibules'. The linear growth of the alga is now terminated. Each outgrowth emits two evaginations, one in the horizontal plane, the other parallel to the axis: the former increases considerably in volume to give rise to the radial chambers of the cap, the latter becomes a part of a ring which encircles the axis subjacently to constitute what is called the inferior corona (Fig. 3). On each of the protuberances of the superior corona two or three hairs appear; they are formed in the usual way though often being incomplete in their development. These morphogenetic events lead to the production of a disk about 1 cm in diameter, containing radial tightly compact chambers, the whole organ finally becoming more or less externally calcified. The number of radial chambers, sometimes called rays, varies from forty to a hundred; their volume is inversely proportional to their number. Differences pertaining to the culture medium may be responsible for the decrease in the number of compartments, but variations may also be due to hybridisation with incomplete dominance, between samples having few large chambers terminated by a flattened apical zone, and other samples having numerous narrow rays terminated by a convex zone. In each compartment of the cap, rounded cysts of various sizes and shape are elaborated; as many as a hundred may be formed, although smaller numbers are more usual and, very occasionally, a whole compartment may give rise to only one cyst. Normally, each alga bears only one cap: on very rare occasions, *Acetabularia* are found to possess two successive reproductive organs, the more distal, however, being the only one to form cysts. Some weeks after their biogenesis, the caps are shed, either as a whole or after breaking into fragments, and the stalk degenerates. The cysts are gradually set free by the breakdown of the cap.

In culture, in the laboratory, a certain number of anomalies are observed. Among these, the most frequently occurring are those which affect the reproductive cap. For instance, the radial chambers may be incompletely fused together; if this is the case they are large, not situated in the same plane and may even overlap, being one above the other; the algae nevertheless remain fertile. If culture conditions are less favourable, definite malformations such as dichotomy and trichotomy of the stalk occur, as well as a series of immature whorls, the shape of which

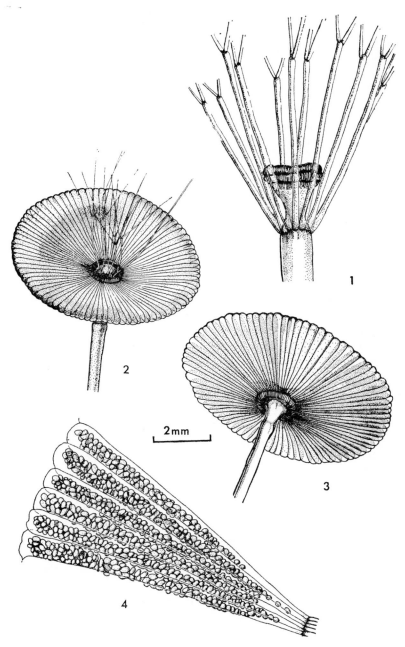

Figure 3. (1) Young cap of *A. mediterranea*. (2) and (3) Adult cap of *A. mediterranea*. (4) External aspect of cysts of *A. mediterranea*.

is something between a hair whorl and a cap; these abortive organs do not form cysts (Dao, 1954a; Bonotto, 1968; Bonotto and Janowski, 1968; Bonotto and Puiseux-Dao, 1970).

The development of *Acetabularia mediterranea* follows a life cycle which has now become classical knowledge: it commences with a latent phase of variable duration, then growth accelerates slightly and becomes much more spectacular. The time required for the plants to become just visible to the naked eye can be almost equivalent to the time they take to pass from this stage to the one at which the stalk and the cap are entirely formed. The maturation of the cysts in the cap is a stationary phase of growth which terminates the life of the alga. Development is characterised by very marked allometry, since the diameter changes from several μ to 0·3–10 mm, whereas the length varies from several μ to about 4–6 cm. The increase in length of the cylindrical axis occurs in a regular way; however, the development of each whorl is followed by a slight arrest in elongation which is more or less marked according to the speed of growth (Dao, 1954a). Very different criteria have been used to evaluate development; the volume is usually calculated from measurements of the length of the axial stalk (Hämmerling and Werz, 1958) and of cell diameter; these authors also use protein content as a way of estimating algal growth. Determination of the wet weight of *Acetabularia* seems to be an accurate criterion, giving a very precise idea of their growth (Shephard, 1965a). In every case, the *Acetabularia mediterranea* studied were 1 cm long at the time of initial measurement. According to Beth (1955a) the increase in height of the axial cylinder follows a linear law, while according to Hämmerling and Werz (1958) growth is an exponential, then linear function of time. Considerable biological variation occurs in fact in *Acetabularia* and with improvements in culture techniques and of methods of measurement, it has become clear that under favourable conditions they continue exponential growth up till the formation of the cap (Shephard, 1955a, Fig. 4).

Acetabularia mediterranea has peculiar features which confer remarkable adaptive ability. If the milieu of culture suddenly becomes unsuitable for growth, only the basal rhizoid survives, while the stalk degenerates; if on the contrary culture conditions are extremely good, the stalks grow more rapidly,

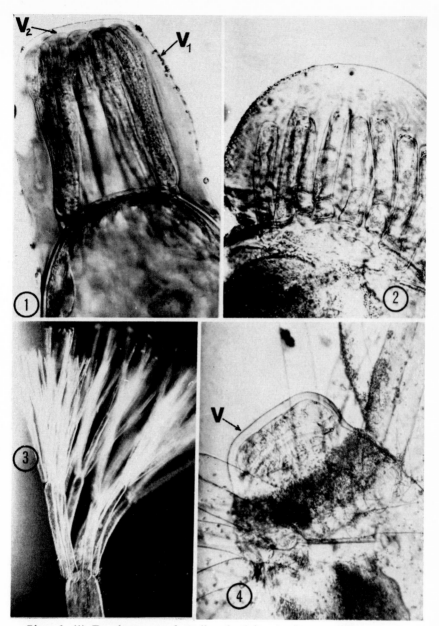

Plate 1. (1) Development of sterile whorl in *A. clavata* under a pectic velum (V_1). At the tips of the primary branches, the second order branches are formed inside small secondary velums (V_2) ($\times 85$). (2) Formation of a sterile whorl under a pectic velum in *A. parvula* ($\times 85$). (3) Sterile whorl of *A. parvula* ($\times 42$). (4) Genesis of a reproductive cap inside a thick pectic membrane (V) in *A. parvula* ($\times 50$). (1), (2) and (4) staining with ruthenium red. (Photo from Valet, 1968.)

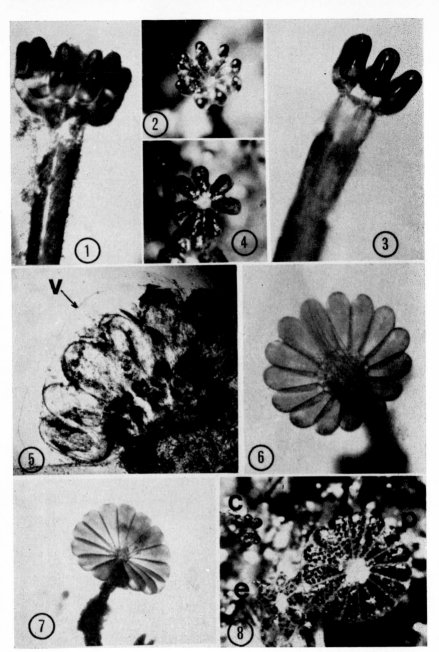

Plate 2. (1) and (2) Formation of a reproductive whorl in *A. exigua* ($\times 30$ and 8). (3) and (4) Development of a cap in *A. clavata* ($\times 8$ and 2·5). (5), (6) and (7) Evolution of the cap in *A. parvula* ($\times 40$, 22 and 15). (8) Reproductive whorls with cysts in *A. clavata* (c), *exigua* (e) and *parvula* (p) ($\times 8$). (Photo from Valet, 1968.)

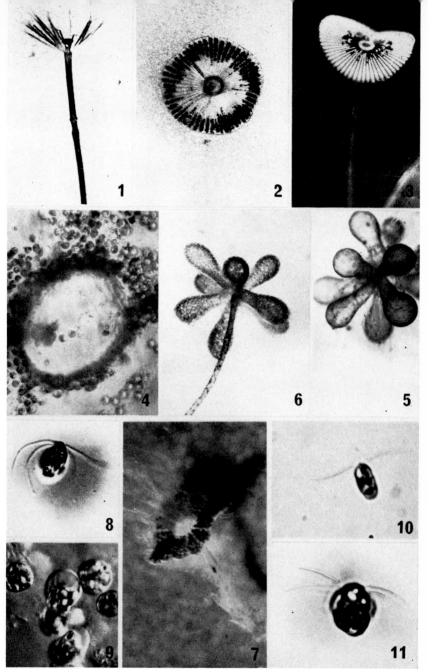

Plate 3. (1), (2) and (3) Young (1) and mature ((2) and (3)) caps of *A. mediterranea* (×2·5). (4) Emission of zoospore in a strain of *A. mediterranea* collected at Salses (×200). (5) and (6) Maturation of cysts in *A. peniculus*: (5) 'White spot' stage. (6) Ripe cysts (×3·7). (7) to (10) Different modes of reproduction in *A. wettsteinii*: (7) Cap containing cysts (×4·3). (8) Quadriflagellate zoospores. (9) Germination of zoospores. (10) Biflagellate gamete. (11) Fertilisation (×1,300). (After Puiseux-Dao, 1962, 1965 and Valet, 1969.)

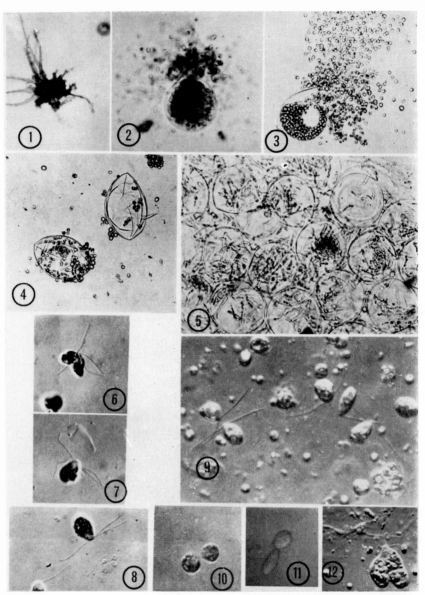

Plate 4. (1) Direct germination of cysts in *A. dentata* (×9). (2), (3) and (4) Emission of zoids in *A. exigua*. The residual vacuole is shown in (3) (×130). (5) Germination (probably asexual) of zoids in *A. clavata* (×160). (6), (7) and (8) Gametes, copulation and zygote in *A. exigua*. (9) and (10) Gametes of *A. clavata*. (11) Gametes in *A. exigua* (×900). (12) Fertilisation in *A. clavata* (×1,000). (Photo from Valet, 1969.)

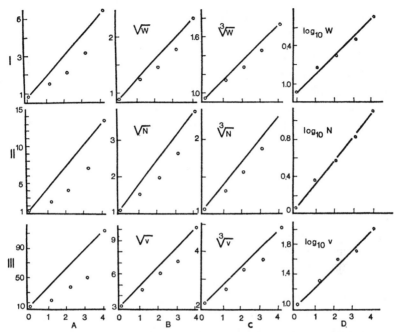

Figure 4. Growth and development of the plastids in *A. mediterranea*. *Abcissa*: time in weeks. *Ordinate*: (I) Weight of the algae in mg. (II) Number of plastids in millions. (III) Volume of the plastids in mm³/1000. *Graphs*: (A) Overall findings. (B) and (C) Ordinates expressed in square or cubic roots. (D) Ordinates expressed in log form. The linear form of the graphs D joining the experimental points (D) suggests that the growth of the alga as well as the increase in number and volume of the plastids, is exponential (After Shephard, 1965a.)

produce sterile whorls, then the reproductive cap. Several periods of dormancy may occur in the same alga, without producing any loss of fertility. Observations carried out in nature, or on tufts of *Acetabularia* brought into the laboratory, show that, at least in poor ecological conditions (brackish water, for instance) the algae may fail to form a cap even after a good season's growth. They then pass the winter in a form in which morphology is limited to the rhizoid plus the base of the axial stalk which will regenerate a new, complete, stalk the following spring. The presence in harvested tufts of three types of plants having reached a finite stage of development, in these poor conditions, suggests that the algae may sometimes take three summers to reach maturity.

2. Morphology and morphogenesis in other Acetabularia

The general behaviour of the different species of *Acetabularia* is remarkably similar; they can, however, be subdivided into two groups, one possessing an inferior corona, the other not. The first subdivision, *Acetabularia sensu stricto*, includes the largest members, surpassing 4 to 5 cm in height; they have only one cap, except in the species *crenulata*, which forms several caps, often separated by sterile whorls. Members of the second sub-group, the *polyphysa*, are small, about 1 cm high, except for *Acetabularia peniculus*, which is much bigger (4 cm) (p. 35).

In all those species which have been observed, development begins in the same way: initially spherical, the young plant rapidly becomes cylindrical, showing very definite apical growth; rhizoids are produced at the opposite extremity. The axis elongates and produces sterile whorls, ten or more in the first group, only a few, five at most, in the second (Valet, 1969). The external cell wall is smooth and as a rule calcified, though in a few of the small species, like *Acetabularia möbii* it folds into ridges. In *Acetabularia polyphysoides*, calcification does not always occur. The hairs develop in exactly the same way as in the *mediterranea* species in all the *Acetabularia sensu stricto* and in *Acetabularia peniculus* (Fig. 5); on the other hand, as far as the *polyphysa* are concerned (Valet, 1969) the sterile whorls are formed in the same way, but on the inside of the apical cell wall of the alga. Indeed, the external part of the latter forms a very fine pellicle* which can be stained with ruthenium red (Fig. 6). Hair rudiments develop beneath this envelope, and so do the succeeding branches; the latter are very close together, and often become entangled. During their formation and growth they gradually distend and rupture the fine protecting membrane; the whorl then spreads freely. The careful observer notices that each time branches are formed they develop beneath similar, ephemerous, sheath-like membranes.

The formation of the reproductive cap is announced by the appearance of a ring of small swellings around the tip of the alga. Differential growth of these gives rise, in the case of *Acetabularia sensu stricto*, to three compartments: the upper and lower of these remain small and form the superior and

* *A. myriospora* never forms sterile whorls (Valet, 1968).

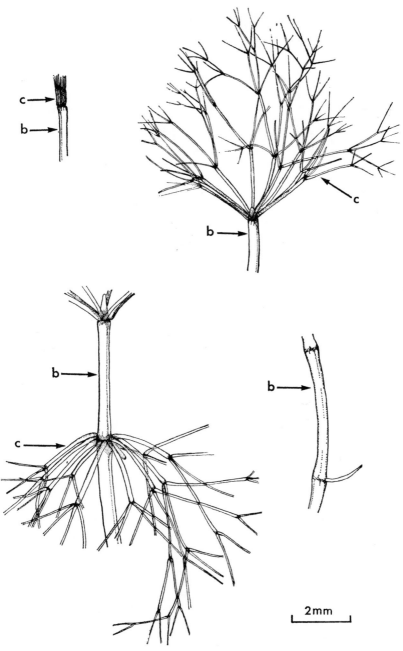

Figure 5. Formation and deciduation of the hairs in *A. peniculus* (left to right):
(b) axial stalk; (c) hair whorl.

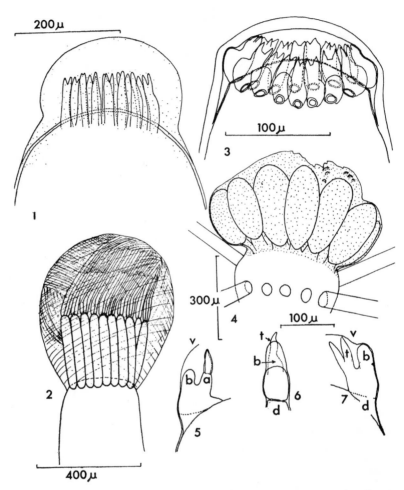

Figure 6. Formation of hairs and of a reproductive cap under a pectic velum in *A. parvula*. (1) and (2) Development of sterile whorl, the hairs of which remain folded up inside the pectic velum for a long time. (3) and (4) Formation of a reproductive cap underneath an initially thick pectic velum (3) which afterwards becomes thinner and breaks, before cap formation is terminated. (5), (6) and (7) Genesis of the chambers of the cap (side view and front view). (a) superior corona; (b) reproductive chamber; (t) rudiments of hairs; (d) vestibule; (v) velum. (After Valet, 1968.)

inferior corona, respectively; the middle chamber increases considerably in size and will contain cysts which are more or less rounded, according to the species. A single cap usually contains more than forty such chambers in algae of this group. Branches or hairs may occur, but are only formed on the superior corona. The *polyphysa* differ from the above described algae in possessing only two initial compartments formed from

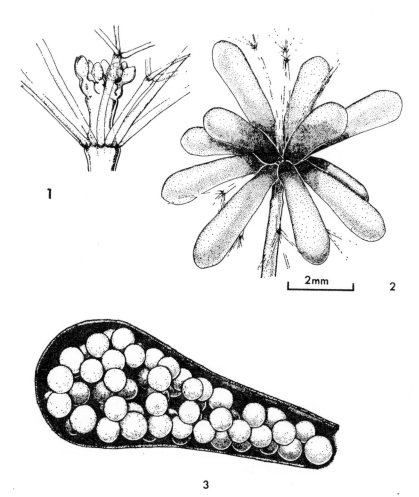

Figure 7. (1) and (2) Formation of a reproductive cap in *A. peniculus*. (3) Cysts of *A. peniculus* within the reproductive cap.

each swelling (since they have no inferior corona); radial cyst-bearing chambers are less numerous also. Moreover, in this group, with the exception of *Acetabularia peniculus* (Fig. 7) the reproductive cap initiates its development within the thickening membrane rich in pectic compounds* which covers the apex. During the growth of the cap the pellicle stretches, becomes thinner, then breaks, though remnants of it often remain (Fig. 6; Plates 1 and 2).

When cultured, all the known species of *Acetabularia* seem to display peculiar features similar to those shown by *Acetabularia mediterranea*: unfavourable conditions produce morphogenetic anomalies; they can survive in latent form and are able to regenerate a stalk and a fertile cap as soon as the medium becomes suitable. Development has been very carefully followed in the case of *Acetabularia crenulata* (Beth, 1955a; Terborgh and Thimann, 1964, 1965). Measurements made by the latter and based on variations in volume, suggest that in the best conditions, growth of the alga occurs exponentially from the time when the stalk is 5 mm long up till the formation of the cap which is usually single in these experiments. These results concord with those obtained by Shephard (1955a) with *Acetabularia mediterranea* and which enabled him to conclude that the development of *Acetabularia* is a very regular process, right up to the time when the cysts are formed in the reproductive caps which have attained their maximum size.

B. THE REPRODUCTION OF *ACETABULARIA*

1. The reproduction of Acetabularia mediterranea and its variations

The development of *Acetabularia*, which lasts six months from the initial germination to the fertile plant, is terminated by the formation of the reproductive cap. In the main, the latter is composed of the large radial chambers (sometimes called 'rays') in which almost all of the protoplasm of the alga accumulates; their contents break up into rounded masses approximately 50 μ in diameter, which become surrounded by a thickened

* 'Pectic velum'.

membrane and are then called cysts. By the destruction of the cap, the cysts are freed and are dispersed by sea currents in nature. This is the first phase of dissemination, which is followed by another. Indeed, after a few months of sluggish life, the protoplasm of the cysts divides to produce biflagellate elements of pyriform shape, which are highly active. These zoids emerge from the cysts, which burst open by means of readily observable lids (Fig. 8; Plate 3). Described as early as in 1877 by de Bary and Strasburger, these zoids measure 2 to 3 μ in width and 5 to 8 μ in length and bear a more or less well-defined eye-spot; they were described isogamous gametes by the latter while no sexuality was observed by the latter. Whatever may be the case, the zoids are positively phototactic at first, then negatively: they then lose their flagellae and round off, to become attached and to transform into young seedlings like those which gave rise to the mature algae from which the cysts came. The life cycle is thus very simple; but even when research on *Acetabularia* was only just beginning, the question was asked whether at cyst level, both sexual and asexual reproduction might persist. The German school, with Hämmerling (1931, 1932), observed that in their cultures, equal sized gametes fertilise one another, but that parthenogenetic development also occurs. In other cultures, on the other hand, reproduction is often asexual, by way of zoospores, as suggested by caryological observations (Puiseux-Dao, 1962). Gametes structure and fertilisation were studied with the electron microscope by Crawley (1963, 1966a,b, 1970).

In fact, culture conditions seem to determine the mode of reproduction. In certain, ill-defined conditions, the latent period of the cysts is shortened and may only last about fifteen days, or even less, while gametogenesis is often short-circuited. In such cases the cysts produce less numerous but bigger zoospores, or may even start germinating themselves, to form a little plant, though this is rare in *Acetabularia mediterranea*. Very exceptionally, in a few rather prolific algae, the stalk, as well as the cap, may be full of cysts and direct germination of the latter may be frequent. Occasionally, too, fragments of cytoplasm remaining in the stalk are directly transformed into plants. The conditions of life of the algae are certainly not the only factors governing their mode of reproduction. Geographical races or

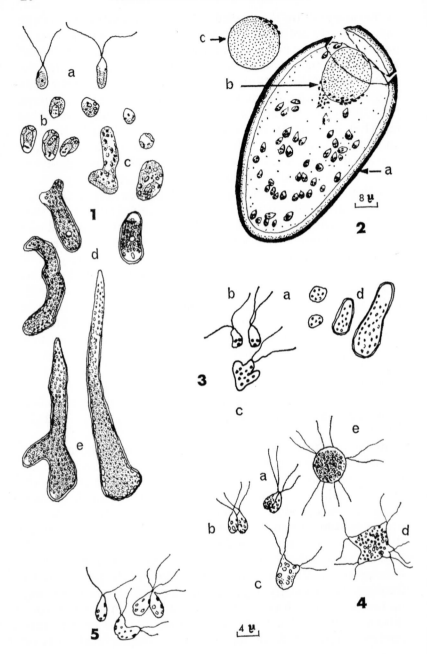

8 μ

4 μ

clones developing at variable rates and possessing diverse more or less stable forms of sexuality, probably exist.

At present, the evidence permits the conclusion that *Acetabularia mediterranea* reproduces sexually by gametes formed in the cysts, each cyst supplying zoids of only one sex. Fertilisation is usually isogamous (Hämmerling, 1931, 1932), sometimes anisogamous, as, for instance, in one brackish water species (Puiseux-Dao, 1962). The alga also multiplies asexually by aid of zoospores elaborated in the cysts as well. Little plants which derive from direct germination of the cysts are also known to occur, though rarely, in this species. The development of these algae depends on culture conditions and also, insofar as the initial speed of development is concerned, on the amount of cytoplasm present in the germinating plant.

2. *The reproduction of other Acetabularia (Plates 3 and 4)*

In this field, two categories of observations are included, according to whether they are made on algae collected in nature, or on algae cultured for several generations in the laboratory. Sexual reproduction identical to that found in *Acetabularia mediterranea* has been described in the following species:

Acetabularia crenulata: Hämmerling, 1943a
Acetabularia schenckii or *Acicularia schenckii:* Beth, 1943a
Acetabularia wettsteinii: {Hämmerling, 1934a,b
{Puiseux-Dao, 1965
Acetabularia exigua: Valet, 1969
Acetabularia clavata: Valet, 1969

In every case, whether in the ovoid cysts (*Acetabularia major*) or in the very regularly spherical ones (*Acetabularia peniculus, Acetabularia wettsteinii*), the cytoplasm breaks up into biflagellate zoids which escape by way of the lid when it

---

Figure 8. Mode of reproduction in *A. mediterranea*. (1) (a) to (e): zoids and germination of zoids (after de Bary, 1877). (2) (a) cyst producing zoospores; (b) and (c) lipid vesicles and carbohydrate granules (after Puiseux-Dao, 1962). (3) (a) and (b) zoospores; (c) zoospores remaining united; (d) direct germinations of zoospores (after Puiseux-Dao, 1962). (4) (a) and (b) isogamous fertilisation; (c), (d) and (e) fertilisation in aggregates (after Strasburger, 1877). (5). Isogamous fertilisation (Puiseux-Dao, unpublished).

opens. Their size varies from 2–4 μ to 6–10 μ, according to the species; it is often difficult to verify the presence of the eye spot, owing to carotenoids occurring as free or as intraplastidal granules. After a period of active, swimming life, isogamous fertilisation occurs between gametes which usually seem to derive from different cysts. The zygotes germinate and give rise to algae resembling the original plants, parents of the cysts. In some species, the cysts have no latent period (*A. wettsteinii, A. exigua, A. clavata*) whereas in others, there is a period of dormancy varying from several weeks to several months (*A. crenulata, A. peniculus*).

Just as in the different cultures of *Acetabularia mediterranea*, this mode of reproduction is subject to a certain number of variations: cases of parthenogenesis have been most often described by German authors (Hämmerling, 1934a,b; 1943a, 1944; Beth, 1943a). Anisogamous fertilisation has been described in one strain: *Acetabularia möbii*, by Nizammuddin (1964). Finally, in *Acetabularia wettsteinii*, asexual multiplication by quadriflagellate zoospores has been observed by Puiseux-Dao (1965).

In the main, it may therefore be said that *Acetabularia* reproduces sexually by way of isogamous gametes formed in the cysts; since these observations are not, however, so very numerous, further study may eventually reveal sexual types of reproduction of a different nature in some species, or, perhaps, its complete suppression in certain species, at least in culture.

C. CULTURE PROBLEMS IN *ACETABULARIA*

The marine Chlorophycea are not easy to culture in the laboratory, probably because our knowledge of their life conditions is still incomplete. Sea water to which nitrates, phosphates and earth extracts have been added ('Erdschreiberlösung' or ESL) has long been known to be the best medium of culture. This medium, the composition of which is unknown, and which may vary according to the origin of the sea-water or of the earth extract, is not very satisfactory; but up till now green algae have seemed to be refractory to long cultures in synthetic media, which do not permit normal development.

Culturing cells, tissues or organs always requires a certain amount of precaution to be taken to avoid infection, and for the choice of nutritive media. These problems will be treated first, while the influence of physical factors, especially light, will be treated in the second part of our study.

1. Culture techniques

Recently, improvements in culture techniques have been made by: Lateur (1963), Puiseux-Dao (1963), Keck (1964) and Shephard (1969). They are based on the early work of Hämmerling (1931) and Beth (1953a).

(a) CULTURE MEDIA

The basic medium corresponds to the classical ESL: sea water, 1,000 ml; $NaNO_3$, 0·1 g; Na_2HPO_4, 0·02 g; earth extract, 50 ml.

The earth extract is prepared in the following way: 100 to 300 g of sieved earth, dried in an oven at 60°C if possible, is added to 1 litre of distilled water. Not every kind of soil is suitable; some soils may give quite toxic concoctions. Florists compost or 'heather' soil may also be used. The mixture so obtained is gently boiled for one and a half to two hours, and is then autoclaved at 120°C for about ten minutes. The cooled supernatant is filtered and kept in the refrigerator; if it has to be kept for several days, the extract is sterilised in the autoclave in small bottles, on two separate days, with an intervening period of twenty-four hours at 37°, to ensure sterility. Controls may be achieved at 37° on gelose. Lateur (1963) recommends the following composition: sea water, 100 ml; glucose, 2 g; nutrient broth, 0·8 g; agar, 2 g.

ESL has been amended in the following way: the amount of earth extract added can be reduced to 0·1 ml instead of 50 ml/l of sea water, suggests Lateur (1963), who uses a very highly concentrated extract. Gibor and Izawa (1963) replace sodium nitrate by potassium nitrate and disodium phosphate by monosodium phosphate. Lateur adds sodium bicarbonate (0·025 g/l). Gibor and Izawa even add glucose and tryptose.

When the development of *Acetabularia* in pure sea water is compared to that of the alga in sea water to which phosphates and nitrates have been added, or ESL, it is found that the earth extract is much more efficient than NO_3^- and PO_4^{---} ions. Ammonium salts are toxic for these algae, whereas the addition of amino acids (0.5 to 1 dg/l) or even asparagine or glutamine amides (1 to 5 g/l) may result in improved growth (Puiseux-Dao, 1962). This would suggest that factors required for the assimilation of nitrates (vitamins for instance) are only synthesised to a slight extent, or not at all, by the algae. This hypothesis should be considered in comparison with the results of Provasoli et al. (1957), who have shown that the B vitamins should be added to the culture media for marine algae.

A few attempts have been made to grow *Acetabularia* in purely synthetic media, but this has proved very difficult: the plants often form stalks lacking whorls, with severely disturbed morphological features (Puiseux-Dao, 1963). In 1964, however, Keck obtained good results with the RILA MARINE MIX (Utility Chemical Company, Paterson, New Jersey) to which nitrate and phosphate had been added. But, unfortunately, he gave no information as to the duration of the trials nor about the aspect of the adult algae. More recently still, Shephard (1969) has described perfectly normal development and morphogenesis of *Acetabularia* grown in an artificial medium rich in microelements and vitamins.

(b) TIME SEQUENCE OF CULTURES

In order to start cultures from *Acetabularia* harvested in nature, reproductive caps containing cysts are generally collected. When algae are transferred from one laboratory to another, this is also the best stage at which to transport them. Indeed, the cysts of the two most studied species (*Acetabularia mediterranea* and *Acetabularia crenulata*) normally last several months or even a year or more. However, the healthier the culture, the shorter is this dormant period, which may even be lost. Strains having a short dormant period may of course have been progressively selected in different laboratories. Whatever may be the normal duration of the dormant period, reproductive caps of species showing dormancy should be kept in the dark and, if possible, at a low temperature (about 6 to 16°C); they are exposed to light for twelve hours a month to avoid the degeneration which may set in if they are kept too long in the dark.

In order to obtain zoids, various techniques are suggested for the *Acetabularia* studied. According to Lateur (1963), Puiseux-Dao (1963) and Keck (1964), it is essential to keep the cysts in the dark for eight days or more, to ensure their maturation. However, if they receive an osmotic or thermal shock at the same time as they are returned to the light, the number of zoids emitted is increased considerably. Hämmerling (1934d) recommends treating the cysts for a few minutes in distilled water, whereas Lateur slightly heats them. In each case, when the caps are cut into little pieces to facilitate the liberation of the zoids, a cloud of flagellate elements showing positive photo-tactism, is obtained within a few (two to fifteen) days. The zoids are then generally divided out into sterile flasks, using sterile pipets. Gibor and Izawa (1963) and Lateur (1963) advise wrapping the culture flasks in black paper for twenty-four hours to prevent phototactism and to encourage uniform distribution of germinations.

Fragments of caps covered with epiphytes, Bacteria and Protophytes can be eliminated by retransferring the zoids, so that the young plants can develop in a clean medium. Infection can be counteracted by treating the young cysts very rapidly, during the period of storage, with 70% alcohol (Puiseux-Dao, 1962) or with different antibiotics (Gibor and Izawa, 1963; Lateur, 1963; Shephard, 1969). Lateur suggests that the freshly collected caps should be treated as follows:

(1) Shake the reproductive caps in a conical flask containing sterile sea water, in the presence of a small brush which has been sterilised in boiling water.

(2) Treat for twenty-four hours in the dark, at 20°C, with the following sterile solution: distilled water, 100 cm^3; teepol (detergent), 1 cm^3. The cysts should then be brought back slowly to normal seawater, in order to avoid bursting the cysts.

(3) Treatment for two to five days, in the dark, in the following solution: pure sea water, 100 ml; mycostatine, 1,000 units/ml; neomycine, 1%.

(4) Stocking of caps at 12°C, in the dark, in sterile sea water, renewed every month.

Gibor and Izawa (1963) have obtained pure cultures of *Acetabularia* by treating the caps in a much more drastic way; after one to two hours immersion in a solution of 10% argyrol (silver-protein), the caps are left for five days in sterile sea water containing antibiotics: Streptomycin sulphate, 200 mg; Penicillin, 100 mg; Mycostatin, 20·000 units; Chloramphenicol, 20 mg; Neomycin, 20 mg; sea water, 5 cm³. Shephard also gives a very complete list of antibiotics and bacteriostatic reagents which are efficient and which can be used to wash the caps (in press).

The young germinating plants obtained from the cysts measure several millimetres after one or two months of culture. They are usually stocked in this stage, being kept in the dark at 16°C and only exposed to light for twelve to forty-eight hours per month; this is, in fact, absolutely essential in the case of species without a dormant cyst stage. They can then be used according to experimental needs. With this procedure it is possible to obtain a given quantity of algae, at will, without having to wait for an emission of zoids, which does not always succeed (when the cysts are too old, for instance). Moreover, when the algae are needed, the initial period of slow growth, particularly susceptible to infection and of variable duration, can be avoided. It should be mentioned that at all stages of their life cycle, *Acetabularia* can support antibiotic treatment (Gibor and Izawa, 1963; Puiseux-Dao, 1963).

When *Acetabularia* are required for experimental purposes, instead of keeping them all together, as was the case for the initial germination, they are divided into groups of thirty to 150 in 200 ml of liquid in dishes or sterile conical flasks. Development can be improved by bubbling through compressed air (Lateur, 1963), but a more useful procedure consists in the frequent renewal of the culture medium, which helps to avoid infection as well as providing sufficient aeration. The cultures can also be gently shaken on a mechanical stirrer for conical flasks, though the medium often forms crystals in this case. In general, the nutritive solutions are changed, insofar as this is materially possible, every fifteen days or every month for basic cultures, every eight days or more frequently during experimental periods.

In order to avoid infection to a maximum extent, Gibor and

Izawa (1963) have even cultured *Acetabularia* without changing either glassware or media from the stage zoospore or zygote through to the 2 cm germling, using very rich nutritive solutions which provide adequately for the early development of the algae: sea water, 900 ml; distilled water, 100 ml; earth extract, 10 ml; KNO_3, 75 mg, sterilised by autoclaving. The following ingredients are then added aseptically: K_2HPO_4, 15 mg; glucose, 500 mg; tryptose (Difco), 500 mg; pH adjusted to 7·5 with sterile K_2CO_3. The richness of the medium makes micro-organisms grow rapidly, and sterility is thus easily controlled; contaminated flasks are eliminated immediately. Such a treat-ment, though well calculated, is not suitable for every type of experiment. Indeed, the metabolism of the plant, and particu-larly that of its plastids, may be abnormal in the presence of glucose, so it would at least be necessary to control their ultrastructure.

2. Culture conditions

Usually, *Acetabularia* are cultured in ESL at a temperature averaging 18 to 25°C, with an alternating light/dark rhythm of 12/12 hours, the light source supplying, 1,000 to 3,000 lux (very approximately 300 ft-ca*).

Few experiments have concerned temperature, since these algae come from warm seas and grow little, or not at all, at temperatures below 18°C. Conversely, bacterial contamination is another danger at too high a temperature.

In fact, even when contamination is limited, temperatures higher than 30° are noxious; the plastids of *Acetabularia* become yellow and the membrane strongly calcified. On the other hand, below 10°C growth is stopped and the protoplasm of the alga contracts within the siphon, where it remains in a dormant state until conditions become favourable again.

The effects of light have, on the other hand, been studied on several occasions. The choice of criteria permitting an accurate estimation of light effects is important and difficult in this type of work, which perhaps explains the lack of agreement of the various experimental results. In fact, changes in illumination modify both the growth and the morphogenesis of the alga.

* ft-ca = foot-candles.

Moreover, double phenomena have to be studied independently, one being the influence of the *amount* of light received, the other the *photoperiodicity*.

In relation to the amount of light, early observations revealed that up to a certain light intensity, the speed of growth is proportional to the degree of illumination, but at higher intensities growth remains constant or may even, on occasions, tends to diminish. At temperatures of 22–24°C, and a daily light period of twelve hours and when *Acetabularia* is cultured in ESL, the following observations have been made (Puiseux-Dao, 1963): when the light source is very weak (from 100 to 200 lux), growth is almost nil. Development remains very slow below 500 lux, and the plants form very few sterile whorls and no reproductive organs; the axial stalks may reach a length of 12 cm, whereas normal fertile algae measure about 4 to 5 cm. The formation of reproductive caps becomes possible between 800 and 1,000 lux. The influence of light on the morphogenesis of different *Acetabularia* can also be observed in nature. It has been analysed by Beth (1953a, 1955a,b) on different species (*Acetabularia mediterranea, crenulata, schenckii, polyphysoides, wettsteinii*). This author used three different types of illumination: weak (600 lux); average (2,500 lux); strong (5,000 lux); quantitative variations were obtained in these experiments simply by varying the duration of the light period each day, from one to twenty-four hours. Increase in length was taken as a criterion of development, plus a few measurements of diameter; the time of appearance of the first cap was considered as a starting point to evaluate morphogenesis. The algae studied generally measured about 1 cm at the beginning of the observations. Various experiments carried out on nucleate and anucleate algae, led Beth to conclude that:

(i) The more light energy they receive, the more quickly *Acetabularia* grow, the more rapidly they form fertile caps, and the shorter are the stalks which carry them.

(ii) Three factors dominate development: the lengthening of the stalk (elongation) the morphogenesis of the cap and the division of the nucleus leading to the formation of cysts.

More light is required for the formation of the cap than for stalk elongation. Moreover, since it has been observed that in

Acetabularia schenckii weak illumination for average light periods produces algae lacking caps but which contain cysts in the axial filament, Beth (1955a) thinks that the division of the single nucleus requires *less* light than the genesis of the cap, but *more* than growth (Fig. 9).

	1	2	3	4	5	6
a	f	N	F	N	N	N
b	2h	2h	2h	4h	8h	12h
c	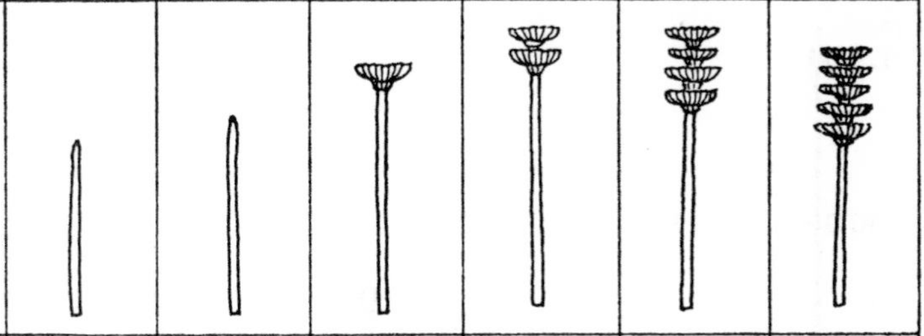					
d	21	24	28	32	32	30
e	0	0	0·8	1·5	3·8	4·9
f	12	18	11	19	17	15
g	2·2	2·4	0·9	1·5	0·6	0·3
h	0·4	1·4	0·7	0·5	0·2	0·3
i	1·0	2·4	0·9	1·7	0·5	0·7
k	3·3	5·6	2·3	3·8	1·4	1·0

Figure 9. The effects of light on *A. crenulata*. (a) Light (f : weak N : normal F : strong); (b) duration of illumination daily; (c) stage of development reached after 72 days culture under varying light conditions, as indicated; (d) length of the algae in mm after 72 days; (e) average number of caps per alga; (f) number of algae studied. (After 72 days, the rhizoids of *Acetabularia* were removed and further development of the anucleate fragments observed under constant culture conditions.) (g) number of sterile whorls formed after amputation; (h) number of caps with a diameter superior to 2 mm formed after amputation; (i) number of caps initiated; (k) total number of new structures. (After Beth, 1953a.)

He emphasises, in his conclusions, the predominating role played by the amount of light received, the photoperiod seeming, in his opinion, to exert no influence. What is more, he emphasised that the life of *Acetabularia* is divided into two distinct phases: the lengthening of the stalk and the formation of the cap.

A much more methodical approach to the study of the effects of illumination is that of Terborgh and Thiman (1964, 1965). In the beginning, they studied the development of tiny plants of *Acetabularia crenulata* under experimental conditions, making sure that, between 5 and 22 mm in length, the increase in volume (expansion) is proportional to the degree of lengthening (extension). They then proceeded to analyse what happens

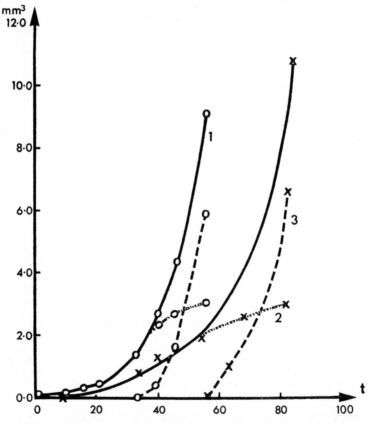

Figure 10. Increase in volume of whole cells (1), of the stalk (2) and of the cap (3) in *A. crenulata* cultured in fluorescent light at an intensity of 300 ft-ca at 25°C; light period: 8 hours (X) and 16h(O) daily. *Abcissa*: time in days. *Ordinate*: volume in cubic millimetres. (After Terborgh and Thimann, 1965.)

in constant light; this enabled them to relate their findings to one single factor, that of light quantity. Thus, it was found that at 25°C, in ESL, the development of the species considered depends a great deal on light between 12 and 55 ft-ca (very approximately 120 to 550 lux). This dependence decreases at higher illumination, and reaches a plateau at from 80 to 100 ft-ca (very approximately, 800 to 1,000 lux) (Fig. 10). In order to focus attention on the photoperiod, they diminished the time of daily exposure to light. When the alternation of light and darkness corresponded to sixteen hours/eight hours respectively, the results obtained, with rare exceptions due to slight varia-tions in experimental conditions, were very similar to those obtained with constant light, and the crucial values given above are very close to those obtained with a photoperiod of 12/12 with *Acetabularia mediterranea*. On the other hand, when the photoperiod is 8/16, the rate of growth is reduced and a plateau is only reached with an illumination intensity of 200 to 225 ft-ca; above this level, even if a light source of very high intensity is used (900 ft-ca for instance) the rate of development is always lower than that of algae living under 16/8 photo-period conditions (even when the latter are only receiving feeble illumination) (Fig. 11). This data provided evidence for

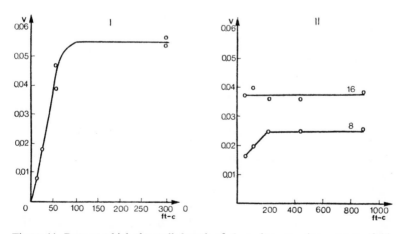

Figure 11. Rate at which the stalk length of *A. mediterranea* increases twofold, as a function of light. (I) In constant fluorescent light (25°C). (II) With 8 and 16 hrs daily light (tungsten or mercury vapour lamps at 23–24°C). (After Terborgh and Thimann, 1964.)

the influence of time of exposure to daylight on *Acetabularia*, whereas, by measuring the increase in length as a function of light, instead of the rate of growth as a function of light, Beth had failed to detect such an effect, although it can be deduced from some of his findings. Moreover, the chlorophyll content of the alga per unit of fresh weight always remains inversely proportional to light intensity, whatever the photoperiod, just as in most plants. Furthermore, for an identical degree of illumination, the quantity of pigment increases if the light period is only slight: at a saturation level of light intensity (225 to 900 ft-ca) *Acetabularia* receiving only eight hours of illumination per day contain fifty to 300 times more chlorophyll than algae receiving sixteen hours of light.

The influence of light on the morphogenesis of the cap in *Acetabularia crenulata* has also been studied by Terborgh and Thimann (1965). Their results, using a source of continuous light, mainly brought confirmation of previous findings. At saturation levels (300 ft-ca, for instance) the algae grow rapidly and produce a fertile cap; the average length of the stalks when 50% of the algae have formed reproductive organs, is found to be 2 to 2·5 cm. With a diminished light source, the stalk may begin to increase in length beyond the first cap, resulting in the formation of a second reproductive organ, generally the only one to form cysts. Low light conditions usually result in a slowing down of growth, defined as a general phenomenon starting with the formation of the young plant and terminating in the production of a cap (page 12): upon the exceptionally long stalks a series of caps successively appear, gradually increasing in size from the lower to the upper part of the stalk. At light levels as low as 12 ft-ca, no reproductive organs are formed at all, while after more than eight months in culture, the stalks measure 8 to 10 cm. An increase in the amount of light is enough to induce cap formation, whereas a reduction in light brings about the degeneration of previously formed caps and slows down the rate of growth of the stalk. Contrary to the opinion expressed by Beth, there does not seem to be any well-defined break in development at the time of appearance of the cap, judging from the study of the growth curves of Terborgh and Thimann, and from the reversibility of morphogenesis described by Dao (1954a) for *Acetabularia mediterranea*.

These data can be summarised according to the schematic diagram proposed by the American authors concerning the control of light on the development of *Acetabularia*, as follows:

Acetabularia crenulata: Terborgh and Thimann (1965)

ht development in ESL at 25°C

$\xrightarrow{\text{-ca}}$ lengthening $\xleftarrow{\text{25 ft-ca}}$ formation of a cap $\xrightarrow{\text{55 ft-ca}}$ ripening of the cap

Acetabularia mediterranea: Puiseux-Dao (1963)

ht development in ESL at 22–24°C

$\xrightarrow{\text{lux}}$ lengthening $\xleftarrow{\text{500 lux}}$ formation of a cap $\xrightarrow{\text{800-1,000 lux}}$ ripening of the cap

The light wavelength received by the algae influences their development considerably (page 115), although initial experiments effectuated by Richter (1962, 1966) failed to supply evidence to this effect. In fact, according to this author, the rate of growth in both *Acetabularia mediterranea* and *Acetabularia crenulata* would be identical so long as they receive the same *amount* of light, whether the wavelength employed is in the red or the blue band. On the other hand, Clauss (1963, 1968) working on *Acetabularia mediterranea* and Terborgh (1965) on *Acetabularia crenulata*, demonstrated that illumination with red light tends to reduce the rate of development first of all, while after a variable delay (two weeks in the *mediterranea* algae, and several days in the other species) growth is almost completely arrested (Fig. 12), the dry weight falls and a concomitant failure to stock soluble sugars is recorded (Clauss, 1968). Furthermore, when the photosynthetic activity of the *Acetabularia* has dropped below levels at which it is detectable, it is possible to restore photosynthetic activity and reinitiate development by placing the algae so-treated in blue light, for short daily periods, even if the latter do not exceed thirty seconds in the case of *Acetabularia mediterranea* (Clauss, 1968) and ten minutes in the case of *Acetabularia crenulata* (Terborgh, 1966). Short exposures to blue light interrupting long periods of exposure to constant red light have similar positive effects, not only on stalk length but also, of course, on dry weight.

Growth, morphogenesis and pigment content of the algae are thus controlled by the amount of light received and by its wavelength; similarly, the photoperiod seems to affect development considerably, and this can be related to the findings concerning the 'biological clock' of *Acetabularia* (page 124).

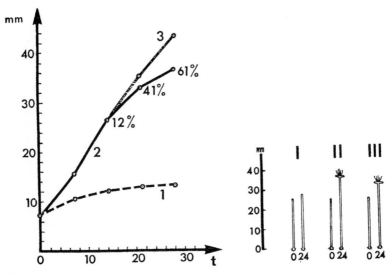

Figure 12. Growth of *A. mediterranea* in red or blue light at equivalent energy levels (4·0 to 10³ erg/cm²). Algae measuring 30 to 35 mm were amputated and the regeneration of the nucleate fragments measuring 5 mm in length, was studied (after 24 hrs rest): (1) continuous red light; (2) blue light. After 14 days, according to the treatment, some cells have formed a cap (2) and some cells lack a cap (3). The percentage of cells having formed a cap is indicated on the right. The aspect of experimental algae: (I) In red light. (II) In blue light. (III) In white light. *Abcissa*: time in days. *Ordinate*: length of stalks in mm. (After Clauss, 1968.)

D. SYSTEMATIC SUMMARY AND CONCLUSIONS

Acetabularia, algae of warm or sub-temperate seas, generally live in shallow, fairly calm water. They are fixed to small pebbles, rocks or shells. The largest species have been known for a long time, whereas a certain number of the smaller species have only been discovered recently. The systematic classification of *Acetabularia* is at present undergoing revision by Valet (1969). In any case, as stated above, *Acetabularia* has been subdivided into two groups which can be distinguished from one another by the presence or absence of an inferior corona. The species so far described are thus grouped as follows:

Sub-group of *ACETABULARIA SENSU STRICTO*
(with two coronas)

Acetabularia mediterranea	*A. crenulata (? A. caraibica)*
Acetabularia ryukyuensis	*A. calyculus (? A. suhrii)*
A. kilneri	*A. farlowi*
A. major	*A. philippinensis*
A. gigas	*A. schenckii (=Acicularia*
A. dentata	*schenckii).*

Sub-group *ACETABULARIA POPYPHYSA* (with one upper corona); all of them are small in size, except for *A. peniculus*

A. peniculus (? A. cliftonii)	*A. polyphysoides*
A. clavata	*A. pusilla*
A. exigua (? A. tsengiana)	*A. myriospora*
A. parvula (? A. moebii,	*A. antillana (=Chalmasia*
? A. Wettsteinii, ? A.	*antillana)*
minutissima)	

Of these species, only a few are used as laboratory material; the most frequently employed are *Acetabularia mediterranea* and *crenulata*; more occasionally, *Acetabularia schenckii*, *moebii* and *polyphysoides* (Beth, 1953a,b, 1955), *Acetabularia major* (Sweeney and Haxo, 1961; page 125) and *Acetabularia peniculus* (Puiseux-Dao unpublished; Plate 8), the last one cultured from living samples sent from Australia by Professor Wormersley (also Schweiger et al., 1969).

Among the small, but little known species, totally unexploited biological material of great value probably exists, having a high rate of growth, and no dormant period.

Structure and ultrastructure of
Acetabularia

The peculiarities of *Acetabularia* cell structure have made this alga a subject of choice for cytological study, although the large water-filled vacuole and more or less calcified cell wall make fixation and embedding fairly difficult.

A. CELL STRUCTURE OF *ACETABULARIA* UNDER THE LIGHT MICROSCOPE (S. Puiseux-Dao, 1962, 1963)

1. General structure of Acetabularia cells

Enveloped in a thick cell wall (10 or more μ in thickness), which is often calcified, particularly in the basal regions of the algae, the *Acetabularia* also possess a huge central vacuole which invades the cytoplasm, itself reduced to narrow parietal bands. These bands are more or less completely filled with numerous small, more or less elongate, chloroplasts (varying from 1 to 2 μ wide to 2 to 8 μ in length).

(a) CELL CONTENT

The giant cell can be sub-divided into three main parts: the rhizoids, the axial stalk, and the apical zone of morphogenesis.

The rhizoids (Fig. 2; page 9) are composed of a group of short extending processes, several millimetres in length, having a very hard, thick wall, which in some species may bear irregular annular ridges (*Acetabularia clavata*). The plastids, present in a relatively abundant cytoplasm, are globular and full of carbohydrate reserves which make them readily stainable with iodo-iodide reagent (brown) or with McManus' stain (pink); they bear some analogy to the amyloplasts of the roots of higher plants. The mitochondria, often punctiform, are not readily visible. One single nucleus is present in one of the rhizoids or at the base of the stalk (2 R = approx. 100 μ); it is a sphere, but so tightly compressed by the vacuole, into which it slightly protrudes, that it is flattened. Within the nucleus the nucleolar mass may be sinuous in shape (*Acetabularia mediterranea*) or, more frequently, be composed of globular agglomerates, of variable size (*Acetabularia crenulata, peniculus*).

The axial stalk also contains, essentially, the central vacuole and the chloroplasts (Fig. 2). The latter are more intensely green and longer than those of the basal rhizoids. One, two, three or even more carbohydrate globules of limited size (2 R $\leqslant$ approximately 1 μ) may be found, as well as small carotenoid crystals. These organelles seem to be arranged linearly in rows which are at the same time affected by the smooth, swift moving cyclotic movements which seem to sweep them along within well defined ribbons of cytoplasm, though individual chloroplasts may actually oscillate around a median point. The mitochondria are always small and very abundant, and usually fairly short. Lipid drops occur to a variable degree, according to the state of the culture; this is also true of grains stainable with anthracene blue which may, according to Stich (1953, 1956a), be meta- or polyphosphates since they readily incorporate large amounts of phosphorus (^{32}P) administered in the orthophosphate form. Angular crystals of a protein nature can also be observed and seem to be intravacuolar; Tandler (1962b,c) attributes a high indol content to them. The internal structure of the hair whorls is exactly the same as that of the stalk; intracellular reserves are negligible, however, while the plastids change in aspect from first to last order ramifications: they become smaller and smaller, and more and more flexible.

The vacuolar system, according to Tandler (1962c) is rich in oxalic and hydrogen ions, as well as in fructosans (du Mérac, 1953), which are easy to observe in the form of spherocrystals after dehydration with absolute alcohol (Puiseux-Dao, 1962). The plastid reserves, which have been analysed from isolated plastids, have been found to contain fructosans (Van den Driessche and Bonotto, 1967).

The apical zone of *Acetabularia*, measuring a maximum of a

few tens of millimetres in length, is relatively poor in plastids. The cytoplasm seems dense, and contains a few mitochondria. A network of special structures which seem to be characteristic of each species (Werz, 1961a) and to contain polysaccharides (Werz, 1960b) is present in this region.

(b) THE CELL WALL

The algae collected in nature are highly calcified (Leitbeg, 1887); in culture, however, when the medium is favourable, calcification rarely occurs. It augments as soon as the medium becomes impoverished, especially in conditions of intense illumination or of high temperature. This membrane is rich in sulphur (Clauss, 1961) and is mainly composed of mannans, according to Miwa (1960), Iriki and Miwa (1960), Mackie and Preston (1967), Frei and Preston (1968). It gradually thickens in the oldest parts of the algae, particularly at the base, where it increases in thickness solely by apposition. At the apex, where the membrane is thinnest, it grows by apposition and by intussusseption (Werz, 1957a). Staining with ruthenium red shows it to be rich in pectic compounds. The appearance of a whorl of sterile hairs is preceded by a ring of tiny convexities around the summit of the stalk, the elongation of which is temporarily arrested. The lysis of the old wall and the biogenesis of membranous substances accompanies the formation of these outgrowths, facts which mainly emerge from the studies of Werz (1966b). As the first branches increase in length, ribbons of cytoplasm migrate into them. The same process is repeated at the summit of the first order branches: lysis of the apical membrane, beneath the wall of the young outgrowth, and migration of cytoplasm into the new branch, as described by several authors (in Bonotto and Puiseux-Dao, 1970). Each time, the morphogenesis of the next order of branches proceeds in an identical manner, so that the anucleate stalks which are formed become shorter and shorter, and poorer and poorer in intracellular substance. The initially communicating channels between succeeding branches are progressively constricted basally and finally closed by obturation with substances staining vitally with ruthenium red. The fine projections from the hairs are transitory, because their bases rupture; the outer-most appendages fall off first (Fig. 2; page 9). In the group *polyphysa*, biogenesis of the whorls occurs under a pectic velum which has been previously described (page 14 and Valet, 1967).

The formation of the reproductive cap, in the species *mediterranea* and, probably, in the other species also, is preceded by annular lysis like a 'necklace of pearls' of the apical membrane (Werz, 1965), which occurs under the membranous outgrowths which will give rise to the superior corona. In their turn, these outgrowths give rise to the radial chambers of the cap (rays), and, if necessary, to the inferior corona. All the radial chambers become filled with cytoplasm, and this apical concentration of the cytoplasm continues to such an extent that the stalk of the algae becomes more and more empty and transparent (Schulze, 1939). A stalk-like internal structure is maintained in the coronas and in the radial chambers, in that there is a large central vacuole; but when the caps begin to mature and the cytoplasm rushes towards the caps, numerous nuclei are observed, originating from the initial single nucleus which has broken down (see page 47). Anomalies in the formation of the cap have been studied in *A. mediterranea* by Dao (1964) and Bonotto (1968) and in different species by Valet (1969).

The chemical composition of the membrane of the stalk has been reported to differ from that of the cap (Zetsche, 1967); both contain mannose, glucose and galactose, but a higher proportion of the latter two sugars is found in the cap, which also contains rhamnose. Finally (Werz, 1967), the synthesis of membrane can be induced by implanting a piece of gelatin into the algal stalk. This author emphasised the role of cytoplasm in the mechanisms which control synthesis of the cell wall (1969).

2. Cytological features of the Acetabularia

(a) THE RESTING NUCLEUS

The nuclei of the different species of *Acetabularia* (Fig. 13 and Plate 5) have often been studied; their aspect, in the very young seedlings measuring about 10 to 20 μ, is perfectly normal; more often they originate from the fusion of two gametes' nuclei, an event which occurs in a classical way (Crawley, 1963, 1966a,b, 1970). They contain a more or less dense network of chromatin, which stains with Feulgen; the spherical nucleolus is basophilic. As the algae grow, the chromatin is less and less readily detectable; specific staining with Feulgen is gradually restricted to the perinucleolar zone, then finally disappears completely; the nucleolar mass, on the contrary, increases considerably in size (Vanderhaeghe, 1957). The observations carried out on two other members of this family, *Batophora oerstedii* and *Cymopolia barbata*, encourage the idea that the nuclei of the Dasycladacea, and probably those of the *Acetabularia*, became polyploid by a series of consecutive endomitoses (Puiseux-Dao, 1962, 1967). The hypothesis may therefore be proposed that *Acetabularia* contains about 14 to 16 times its primitive stock of chromosomes, whereas the nucleolar mass may well represent an association of nucleoli, each corresponding to a normal set of chromosomes. This hypothesis is in contradiction with the classical theory which, since the work of Schulze (1939), holds that the gigantic nucleus of *Acetabularia* is diploid. However, polyploidy in Dasycladales is slight as compared with growth in volume of the nucleus; this might explain the faint Feulgen reaction.

When metabolism is active, the nucleolar mass has very

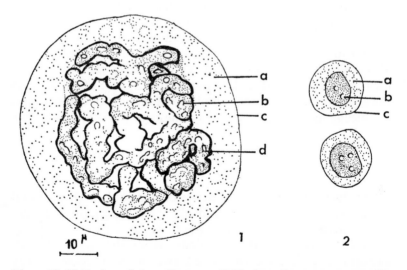

Figure 13. (1) Nucleus of *A. mediterranea*. (2) Nucleus of a very young germling of *A. mediterranea*: (a) nucleoplasm; (b) nucleoli; (c) nuclear membrane; (d) nucleolar vacuole. *Fixation*: Navaschin in sea water; staining with anthracene blue. (After Puiseux-Dao, 1962.)

strong affinity for basic stains (toluidine blue, pyronine, azure blue) or acetic azocarmine (Brachet, 1952; Werz, 1959; Puiseux-Dao, 1962). It is also very voluminous and therefore seems likely to be very rich in RNAs and basic proteins. The nucleoplasm itself is seen to be full of round or ovoid particles which are more or less readily detectable using the same techniques, while the nuclear membrane seems to be bordered by a fringe of such particles on the cytoplasmic side. The latter have been interpreted in *Acetabularia mediterranea* and in *Batophora oerstedii* where they are even more readily observed, as nuclear emissions containing substances of nuclear origin (Puiseux-Dao, 1958a). They have been studied by Werz (1961c and 1962) in normal *Acetabularia* and in isolated nuclei (Plate 6) and probably contain RNAs and proteins.

The nucleus changes in aspect as a function of culture conditions. Nuclear volume has been reported to diminish when the algae are deprived of light (Stich, 1951a). This author has demonstrated that after fifteen days in the dark, the nucleus shrinks and the nucleoli run together into a rounded, only slightly basophilic agglomerate. In addition to these changes in size and stainability, disturbances are observed affecting nuclear emissions, which, while frequent and normal under ordinary light conditions, become rare and extremely variable in the absence of light, a few being eight to ten times larger than in the controls (Puiseux-Dao, 1958b, 1960, 1962a; Hämmerling J. and Ch., 1959; Werz, 1961c, 1962). Such changes in size of the nucleoli and of the nucleus are also found to a greater or lesser extent in algae treated with trypaflavin or with monoiodoacetic acid (Stich, 1951b, 1956b, 1959; Werz 1957d, 1959); inhibitors of oxidative phosphorylation like sodium usnate or dinitrophenol give very similar results, as do streptomycin and uv radiation (Brachet, 1951, 1952; Brachet et al., 1955) as well as beta-mercaptoethanol (Brachet, personal communication). Werz (1957c) adds cobalt nitrate to the list of active substances. Finally, more recently, Brachet, Denis and de Vitry (1964) and Zetsche (1964b) have shown that actinomycin D also provokes, in *Acetabularia*, a loss in nuclear basophilia together with an overall reduction in nuclear and nucleolar volume, the latter organelle sometimes disappearing altogether (Plate 5); puromycin seems to be less efficient. It should be noted that all these changes take place fairly slowly, the final effects being obtained after about two weeks.

The sum of these different observations has led to the conclusion that the single nucleus of *Acetabularia* is metabolically extremely active, one of its functions consisting in the elaboration of complexes of RNAs and proteins which move into the cytoplasm. This hypothesis has been studied in a dynamic way by Brachet's school, using the technique of autoradiography (page 76).

(b) THE APICOBASAL CYTOPLASMIC GRADIENT

An apicobasal gradient can be detected in these algae, using staining *in toto* with basic stains or with acetic azocarmine. The apex, a privileged zone of morphogenesis, stains more strongly than the rest of the cytoplasm, and the intensity of staining decreases progressively towards the base of the siphon. Here again, the nucleolus and the perinuclear region stain very heavily. The young buds of the sterile whorls also stain very intensely, as do the rudiments of the succeeding branches; early morphogenesis of the cap is also marked by intense affinity for such stains (Werz, 1960a). Autoradiographic studies have shown even more clearly the presence of this apicobasal gradient, which is lost when the algae are kept in the dark.

B. CELL STRUCTURE OF *ACETABULARIA* AS SEEN BY ELECTRON MICROSCOPY

1. General structure of Acetabularia cells

It has been possible, using electron microscopy, to check the existence of the structures observed under the light microscope, and to obtain further details. Inside the thick cell wall which is composed of several sheets (Boloukhère-Presburg, 1969), the hyaloplasm is found to be very sparse and to consist of vacuolised bands or ribbons full of plastids. Small areas of the hyaloplasm contain mitochondria having classical structure, and small sized dictyosomes, numerous ribosomes and lipid droplets are also observed. Intravacuolar protein crystals seem to be connected by fine tubular canals to the hyaloplasm and display a regular, loose, geometrical arrangement (Plate 5).

The apex seems to be relatively rich in polysomes (Van Gansen and Boloukhère-Presburg, 1965) and in dictyosomes, especially at the time of morphogenesis of the cap; the latter may well, by virtue of their position, play a part in the synthesis of the apical membrane (Werz, 1965). Special features of algal basal structure are associated with the nucleus and the stock of plastids. Moreover, the nucleus and the plastids of *Acetabularia* have received more attentive study by electron microscopy than any other part of the alga.

2. *Special features of the ultrastructure of the nucleus and the plastids*

(a) THE NUCLEUS

When observed with the electron microscope, using various techniques (Crawley, 1963, 1964; Werz, 1964; Van Gansen and Boloukhère-Presburg, 1965), the nucleus, which is very difficult to embed and cut correctly, presents very special features. It is bounded by a very thin nuclear membrane perforated by nuclear pores and surrounded by a thin layer of cytoplasm which itself sends out buds into the peripheral vacuolar system. The nucleoplasm contains a network of fibrils and of grains which look like ribosomes, as well as tiny, less osmiophilic masses. The well known, voluminous, nucleolar mass, consists of three zones: one is peripheral and is distinctly composed of grains resembling ribosomes, the middle zone is granulofibrillar, whereas the innermost zone, which is clearer in the micrographs, seems to be of fibrillar nature (Plate 7).

The very numerous cytoplasmic blebs which project out from the perinuclear pellicle, are rich in grains resembling ribosomes which therefore look like those seen in the nucleolus. These structures may contain nuclear evaginations; they probably correspond to the nuclear emissions or blebs observed by light microscopy by Puiseux-Dao (1958a) and by Werz (1961c, 1962).

Ultrastructural observations of the nucleus of *Acetabularia* have been relatively rare, because of technical difficulties. However, Boloukhère-Presburg has studied the effects of actinomycin D (1965) and of puromycin (1966) added to the culture medium. While the latter has practically no effect on nuclear structure, actinomycin on the other hand brings about important changes (Plate 7). The main ones are as follows: decrease in nucleolar and nuclear volumes accompanied by fragmentation and, sometimes, complete disappearance of the nucleus, facts which had already been observed with the light microscope (Brachet et al., 1964); segregation of nucleolar material in tiny osmophilic globules; reduction of the granular zone and rarefaction of nuclear buds. The latter changes are certainly related to loss of basophilia and to the reduction in nuclear emissions observed for other inhibitors by light microscopy (page 41).

(b) THE PLASTIDS

Descriptions of the ovoid plastids of *Acetabularia* generally confer upon them a very simple structure. They possess a double membrane which is fairly easy to demonstrate; bundles of peripheral saccules surrounding a stromatic zone. The latter contains one or more carbohydrate granules and more or less abundant osmiophilic granules which are, without doubt, identical to the carotenoid grains seen under the light microscope (Puiseux-Dao, 1963, 1966; Crawley, 1964, 1965; Van Gansen and Boloukhère-Presburg, 1965; Werz, 1964, 1965). The stroma is rich in ribosomes and in fibrils forming a network, the DNA nature of which is shown in Plate 9 (Werz, 1965; Puiseux-Dao, 1966, 1967). Using the technique of Kleinschmidt (Werz, and Kellner, 1968a,b; Woodcock and Bogorad, 1968, 1969; Green et al., 1970), it has been possible to isolate and to spread this network; this DNA is linear or looped, never circular. The plastids found in the basal part of the algae possess very few internal lamellae, and are filled with reserves looking like one, or several adjacent granules which are extremely voluminous (Van Gansen and Boloukhère, 1965). The plastidal population in this basal region seems to become more and more heterogenous as the cell differentiation progresses (Boloukhère-Presburg, 1969; Puiseux-Dao and Dazy, 1970). All the *Acetabularia* have similar plastids (Plate 8); in *Acetabularia killneri*, Rickettsies have been observed in the stroma of the plastids (Puiseux-Dao, unpublished).

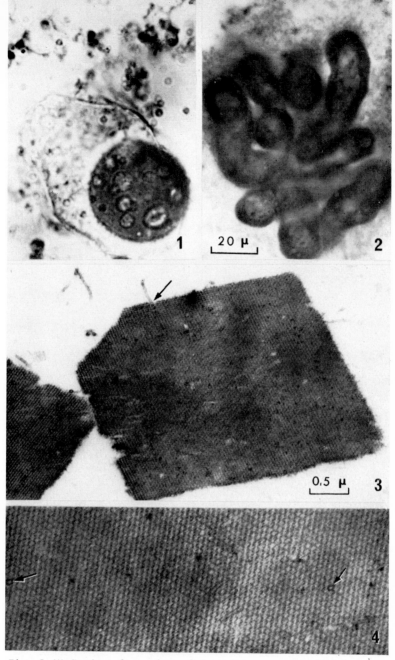

Plate 5. (1) Section of a nucleus of *A. mediterranea* treated with actinomycin D (10 µg/ml). (2) Section of a nucleus of *A. mediterranea*. Fixation: acetic alcohol; staining: methyl green/pyronine. (After Brachet et al., 1964; photos from Brachet.) (3) Protein crystal from *A. mediterranea* detected with the electron microscope as described by Bouck (1964). Such crystals are always associated with the trabeculae limited by a membrane (arrow). (4) Grain of the crystal in which the trabeculae, in section, are visible. (Puiseux-Dao, unpublished.)

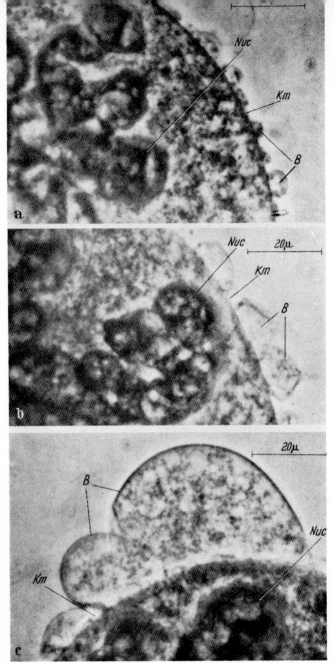

Plate 6. Isolated nuclei of *A. mediterranea*, fixed and stained for (a) 15 seconds, (b) 30 seconds and (c) 1 minute after being isolated. Nuc: nucleolus; Km: membrane; B: blebs. (Photo from Werz, 1962.)

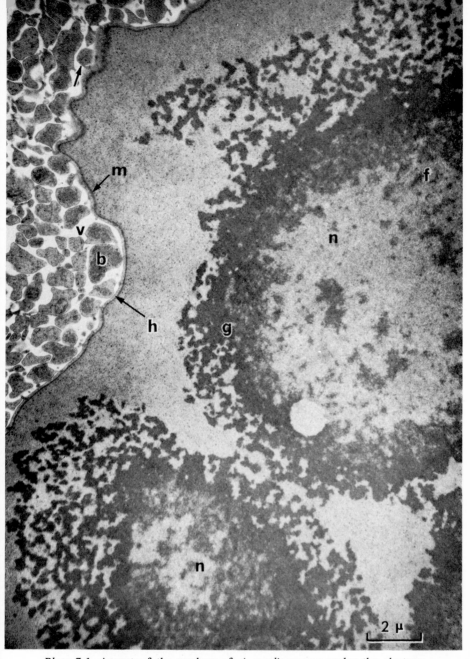

Plate 7.1. Aspect of the nucleus of *A. mediterranea* under the electron microscope. On the right nucleolar fragments (n) are visible; their structure is granulofibrillar (f); around them are clusters of granules (g). The black border around the nucleoplasm is the nuclear membrane (m). The nucleus is surrounded by a very thin hyaloplasmic layer (h) which seems to be juxtaposed to the vacuole (v). The perinuclear buds (b) are comprised of small, dense cytoplasmic masses which are visibly related to the nuclear region (arrow). These probably correspond to the nuclear emissions observed by light microscopy; they sometimes include nuclear evaginations. (Photo from Van Gansen and Boloukhère-Presburg, 1963.)

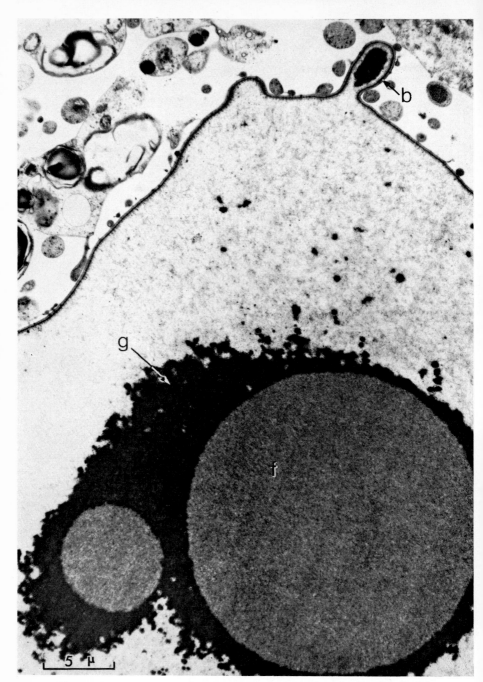

Plate 7.2. The aspect of the nucleus of *A. mediterranea* treated with actinomycin D. Both nucleus and nucleolus are below normal size. The perinuclear emissions (b) are reduced in number and abnormally osmiophilic. The nucleolus comprises a clear central zone (f) and a very osmiophilic peripheral zone (g). (Photo from B018ukhère-Presburg, 1965.)

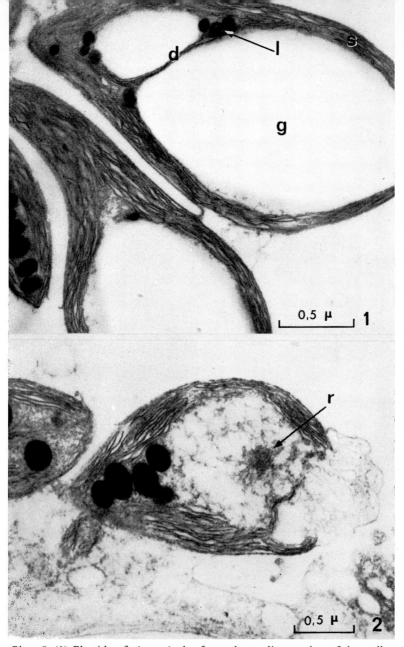

Plate 8. (1) Plastids of *A. peniculus* from the medium region of the stalk. Peripheral saccules (s) surround one or two carbohydrate granules (g). The stroma is very limited, and lipid drops (l) are visible. Between the carbohydrate granules the 'diagonal' lamellae can be seen (d). (2) Plastid of *A. peniculus*, the external membranes of which are slightly ruptured. Such rupture always occurs in the same position; it may be an artefact due to fixation. However, careful comparison of the various types of plastid present in the same stalk suggest that these tears are evidence of healing after the division of the plastid units. In *A. peniculus*, dense granular masses (r) are often visible, resembling a nucleolar type of structure. (Puiseux-Dao, unpublished.)

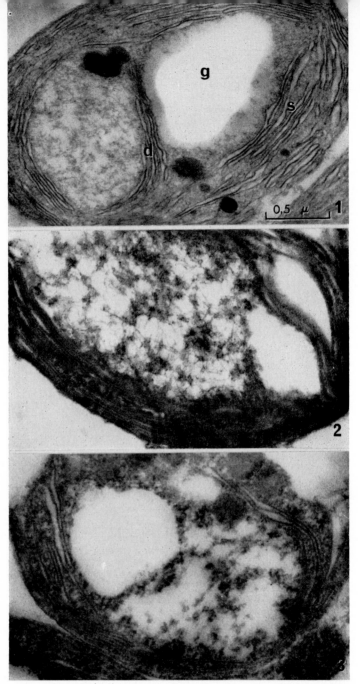

Plate 9. (1) Plastid of *A. mediterranea* made up of two units. Bundles of peripheral lamellae are visible (s) as well as the 'diagonal' lamellae which separate the two carbohydrate granules. Only one of these granules is seen in section (g); the stromatic zone surrounding the other is visible. (2) Evidence for the presence of fibrils of DNA in the stroma between the carbohydrate granules and the saccules. (3) Disappearance of the DNA fibrils of the plastids after treatment with deoxyribonuclease during fixation. (After Puiseux-Dao et al., 1967.)

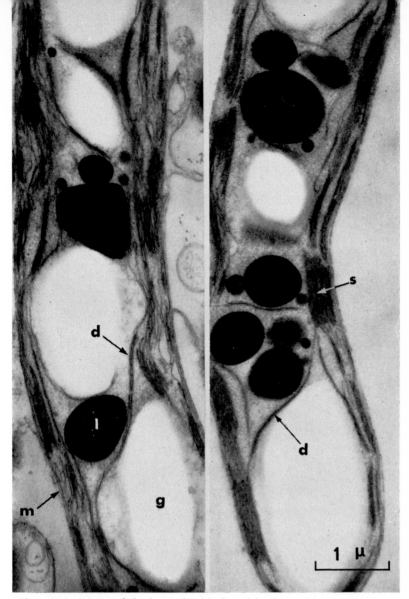

Plate 10.1. Aspect of the long plastids found in the stalks of *A. mediterranea* kept in the dark for two weeks. The external membrane of the plastid (m) is very clearly visible. Large carbohydrate granules are still present (g); between them the 'diagonal' lamellae can be seen (d) as well as large droplets of lipid nature. The peripheral saccules, especially, constitute bundles of tongue-like structures (s).

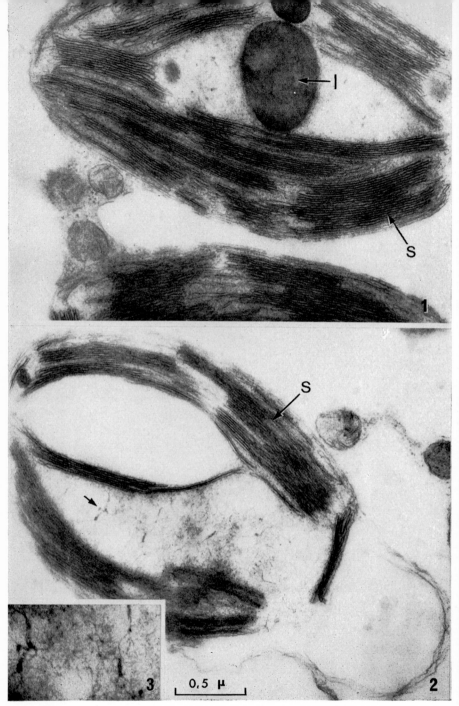

Plate 10.2. The aspect of the plastids observed in the stalks of *A. mediter-ranea* maintained in darkness for five weeks, then illuminated for fifteen minutes only. The plastids often display ruptures thought to be due to the separation of plastid units. Many short lamellae (s) form piles of tongue-like structures of variable size. Big lipid droplets (l) can be seen. In the stroma the DNA looks like a thick cord (3) (arrow). (Puiseux-Dao, unpublished.)

The saccules of the chloroplasts are found to be arranged in a geometrical way. When the plastid contains only one grain of reserve, the latter is surrounded by two groups of lamellae of variable length diverging from the two opposite poles. The saccules adhere to one another in packets of two or three, and may even anastomise. When plastids are isolated in a tris buffer containing saccharose, some of them may burst, showing the saccules to resemble more or less wide ribbons folded upon themselves several times, and united along the borders as if sewn together. This organisation is even easier to see if the isolated plastids are treated with ribonuclease (Puiseux-Dao, unpublished).

A plastid containing two carbohydrate granules always has the following, regular, geometrical pattern (Plate 9): two symmetrical groups of peripheral lamellae surround the storage grains which are abundant when the temperature and the level of light are high. Moreover, diagonal saccules separate the two grains; they occur in two bands, diverging from the two opposite poles of the plastid. In this way, each granule of reserve material is sheathed by packets of elongate lamellae originating at the initial pole of the plastid and converging together in opposite directions in relation to the grain. Thus, a plastid having two carbohydrate granules is composed of two identical units similar to a plastid with one granule. It is usually possible to observe, in plastids having three, four or even more grains of reserve, diagonal lamellae between the granules; it has therefore become possible to assume that the plastids of *Acetabularia* are made up of one or more identical adjacent units (Puiseux-Dao and Dazy, 1970; page 119).

The plastids are organelles in which the lamellar structure is in fact relatively labile; the effects of light, or its absence, and of different inhibitors, have often been studied in different materials.

When *Acetabularia* are left in the dark for at least a week, the plastids become long, thin and less numerous; reserve materials tend to disappear. This is equally visible with a light microscope and an electron microscope (Shephard, 1965; Boloukhère-Presburg, 1969a). The plastids are elongate and up to eight carbohydrate granules can be counted. Under the conditions used (Puiseux-Dao and Dazy, 1970), the latter (Plate 10) though smaller than in algae which receive enough light, are nevertheless clearly visible with the electron microscope, although they do not become visible after staining with the iodo-iodide reagent, under the light microscope. They only disappear completely after seven weeks in the dark. The lamellae look shorter and the external membrane of the plastid is easier to observe than in the controls; however, diagonal lamellae are always present. The osmiophilic granules which are lipid in nature are often very voluminous in such cases and may contain pigments. As soon as the algae are brought back to normal light conditions, new lamellae seem to form very quickly; within fifteen minutes the plastids are full of piles of short saccules, looking like grana (Fig. 10). Later these lamellae increase in length and take on a normal aspect, the units separate and numerous normal sized plastids are once more to be found (page 122).

Puromycin markedly reduces the number of lamellae in the plastids and tends to induce a disordered arrangement of the former. Some of the plastids may not contain any saccule at all, others are found to burst (Bouloukhère-Presburg, 1966). A disordered disposition of piles of short lamellae is also observed with actinomycin (Bouloukhère-Presburg, 1965). The plastids of *Acetabularia* thus react like those of other algae, in which such effects have already been described. They are extremely sensitive, the lamellae are very rapidly affected; they become very short, as is the case when ethionine is administrered to certain *Euglena* (Puiseux-Dao and Levain, 1966) or when *Mougeotia* is treated with ribonuclease (Puiseux-Dao, 1964). They may form piles of saccules having a granum aspect, like those obtained when *Euglena* is treated with streptomycin (Siegesmund et al., 1962) or in some life stages in *Protosiphon* (Berkaloff, 1968).

Although the nuclei and the plastids of *Acetabularia* are found to be the most sensitive organelles from an ultrastructural point of view, it is worth recording a few observations on the effects of more than fifteen days of darkness on the mitochondria and on the distribution of ribosomes in the algae. Werz (1964) has reported the appearance of innumerable lamellae in certain mitochondria. Moreover, Puiseux-Dao (unpublished) has come to the conclusion that the numerous ribosomes present in the hyaloplasmic bands of such algae are actually ribosomes which do not migrate towards the apex, a supposition which would explain the absence of the apicobasal gradient in such algae, as seen from light microscopy. A modification of the apicobasal gradient was also observed for ribosomes by Boloukhère-Presburg (1969a). She also studied the transformations of the plastids during the life cycle of *Acetabularia*, a process which appears to be very complex.

In all the species of *Acetabularia*, cell structure is thus seen to be extremely constant. This is equally true for the nuclear cycles.

C. EVOLUTION OF THE NUCLEI AND NUCLEAR CYCLES IN *ACETABULARIA*

First studied by Schulze (1939) in *Acetabularia mediterranea* and *Acetabularia wettsteinii*, the nuclear cycle has been found to be remarkably similar in the different Dasycladaceae (Puiseux-Dao, 1962a, 1967; Valet, 1969).

1. The division of the single nucleus: the daughter nuclei

The nucleus, which has already been described, is the single nucleus which can be observed in every species of *Acetabularia* from early germination when the alga measures several millimetres in length up till the time when it possesses a cap which is coming to completion. The single nucleus divides when the morphogenesis of this reproductive organ is at an end.

The elaboration of the reproductive cap at the apex of the stalk is preceded by the division of the nucleus into myriads of daughter nuclei and into unused debris. Prior to this event, there is an increase in the size and number of nuclear secretions, visible as small rounded globules in the perinuclear cytoplasm. Within the nucleus of the algae, the nucleoli, when fixed and stained, have less distinct boundaries; the nucleus breaks up into smaller and smaller lobules containing mitotic figures which are normal, apart from their minuteness (Fig. 14). The tiny nuclei (having a diameter of 2μ) resulting from these mitoses continue to divide for a limited period, and are then

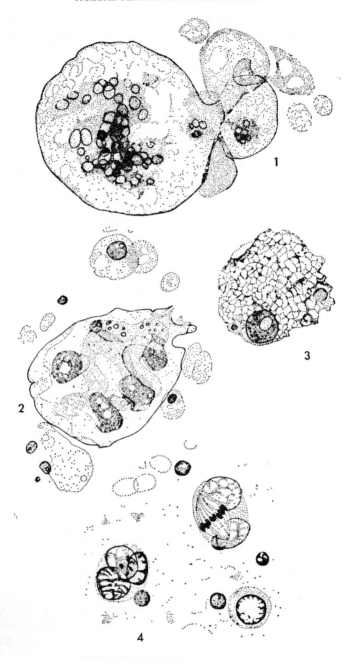

carried towards the reproductive organ by cytoplasmic stream-ing. The site of the original nucleus is usually recognisable by an abandoned, degenerate mass. Division ceases during nuclear migration towards the tip. The nuclei, now in a resting period, are shared out in a regular way within the cytoplasm of the radial chambers of the cap. In the living plant the presence of the nuclei is signalled by a central region of cytoplasm which is devoid of plastids (Plate 3) and which is stained by reagents which are specific for the nucleolus. The increase in size of each nucleus gives them a classical aspect; each contains a single, spherical nucleolus and the peripheral zone disappears, tending to suggest that the cytoplasm probably contributes something to the nucleus at this stage.

Polygonal shaped demarcations now appear in the region of the external membrane of the reproductive organ, between it and the superficial nuclear zone. These polygonal plates form ingrowths perpendicular to the wall of the cap which come to enclose more or less equal areas of cytoplasm and vacuolar sap. Their meeting, in the axial, central region, completes the forma-tion of the cysts. The lid or flap which closes each of the cysts is formed and delimited at the level of the first polygonal thicken-ings (Schulze, 1939; Puiseux-Dao, 1965).

2. Changes in the nuclei of the cysts

Each cyst at first contains only one nucleus with a single spherical nucleolus. Shortly after the formation of the cysts, several mitoses occur within them, until the cyst possesses about twenty to forty nuclei before entering its resting or hibernating period.

Mitoses recommence when zoidogenesis takes place (Fig. 15); they seem to resemble in every way those which occur in the stalk after nuclear division, or in the young cysts. Meiosis has never been observed during the divisions leading to the forma-tion of zoids, except perhaps in one case for the *Batophora*

Figure 14. (1) Vegetative nucleus of *A. wettsteinii*, about to divide (×2000). (2) Vegetative nucleus of *A. mediterranea* undergoing division (×3200). (3) End of the division of the vegetative nucleus of *A. wettsteinii*. Debris not used in the formation of the small daughter nuclei (×1600). (4) Division of the daughter nuclei of *A. mediterranea* (×2900). (After Schulze, 1939.)

(Puiseux-Dao, unpublished) and for *Acetabularia*, Schulze (1939) only describes having observed two, not very convincing, meiotic figures. The primary division of the nucleus, it may be objected, might be a meiotic one, whether the undivided nucleus be polyploid or diploid. We have in fact observed, particularly in *Batophora* which has very large nuclei and in which direct germination of the cysts is frequently observed, that any area of the cytoplasm containing a nucleus is able to grow into a normal adult alga. Parthenogenetic development could occur in such zones, and in the zoids, but insofar as directly germinating cytoplasmic areas is concerned, it is more likely that the nuclei are diploid as in other siphonous Chlorophyceae (Puiseux-Dao, 1967a). Meiosis might occur in a varying number of cysts and produce gametes which copulate, this leads to caryogamy, as observed by electron microscopy by Crawley (1966) and by Woodcock (unpublished). Nevertheless, it is not impossible that some of the gametes develop parthenogenetically as was described earlier by Hämmerling (1934a). Moreover, if the *Acetabularia* nucleus is polyploid, which is possible, it would not seem necessary for gametes containing 'n' number of chromosomes to be produced, and fertilisation might even take place, for instance, between zoids containing 2n chromosomes.

3. The nuclear cycle in Acetabularia

Throughout the Dasycladales, the life cycle is remarkably homogeneous; it is most fully known in *Batophora oerstedii* (Puiseux-Dao, 1962). The same life cycle seems to occur in *Acetabularia*, although sexual reproduction seems to be more frequent for most of them, whereas vegetative reproduction, including the budding out of cysts, is rare. (Diagram on p. 52.)

D. CONCLUSIONS

The *Acetabularia* are at present the best known among the Dasycladales, particularly from the point of view of the cytology and remarkable structural and ultrastructural homology observed among them. These giant cells, containing only one nucleus, which is probably polyploid, differentiate at a cellular level very like higher plants; the upright chlorophyllian stalk terminates in an apex at which morphogenesis and growth occurs, and there is also a basal system of rooting which simultaneously serves as a storage and a survival organ, when conditions of life become difficult (Puiseux-Dao, 1965).

The axial stalk is mainly characterised by its numerous

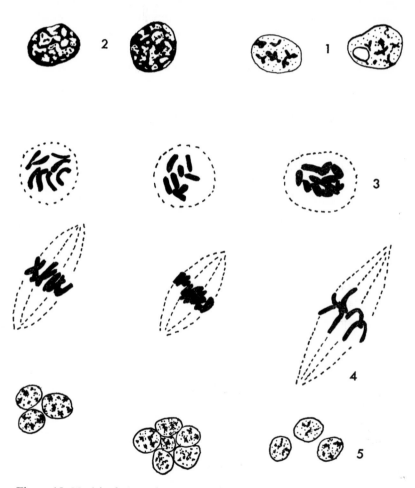

Figure 15. Nuclei of *A. mediterranea* undergoing mitosis in the cysts, during sporogenesis. (1) Nucleus at rest. (2) Prophase. (3) Metaphase plate. (4) Metaphase. (5) Nuclei of the future zoospore, still grouped together. (After Puiseux-Dao, 1967.)

plastids and by its well defined morphology, being composed of one or several adjacent units. The apicobasal gradient in the distribution of basophilic and protein substances, particularly in ribosomes, is also typical. This gradient disappears when the algae are maintained in darkness.

The voluminous nucleus possesses an enormous nucleolar granulofibrillar mass rich in RNAs. Numerous cytoplasmic blebs which project out from the nucleus seem to contain ribosomes. The nucleus, nucleolar morphology, as well as these blebs are very sensitive to life conditions, metabolites, anti-metabolites, inhibitors added to the culture medium.

LIFE CYCLE OF *Acetabularia*

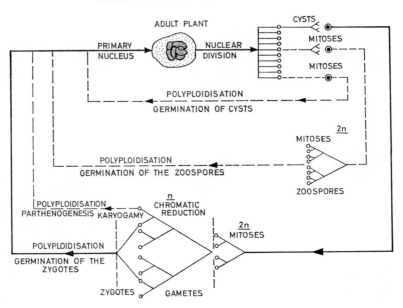

4

Merotomy and grafting

Experimental *merotomy* (sectioning of cells in nucleate and anucleate parts) and grafting, as well as the now very familiar technique of nuclear implantation, have been perfected by the German school.

A. MEROTOMY

Hämmerling first began to concentrate on merotomy experiments and studies of polarity in *Acetabularia* in 1932 and later years, and most particularly in 1934. The single nucleus of the alga is always situated in the rhizoid and only divides when the cysts are about to form. The axial stalk, which may easily reach a height of 4 cm, can easily be sectioned to produce two, three or even more pieces; only the basal fragment contains the nucleus. Each nucleate fragment, even the smallest, limited for instance to the rhizoid, is able to form a complete new alga with its fertile, reproductive nuclei. This is true even when the alga is cut several times, consecutively, whatever the age of the plant. The anucleate portions also survive for several months; when they are big enough and have been obtained from healthy algae, they elongate and produce new whorls, and even one or two reproductive caps, but the latter always remain sterile. Fragments coming from the basal part of the alga differ from those derived from the apex; the latter regenerate more readily, whereas the former have a distinctly lower potential of development, which may be restricted to very slight elongation, or even complete absence of growth. The differing morphogenetic capacities of the nucleate and anucleate fragments are found in all those *Acetabularia* which have been tested from this point of view (*Acetabularia mediterranea, crenulata, wettsteinii*: Hämmerling, 1932, 1934a,b,c, 1935, 1943a, 1946a;

5—AACB * *

schenckii: Beth, 1943a; *peniculus*: Puiseux-Dao, unpublished). They depend, essentially, on the conditions under which the algae are cultured.

On the basis of these results showing that the survival and morphogenetic potentiality of the anucleate fragments are already determined at the time of dissection, Hämmerling advanced the following hypothesis:

(1) Morphogenetic substances of nuclear origin must exist.

(2) The future developmental potentiality of the anucleate fragments depends on the amount of these substances present in them at the time of transection.

(3) There is an apicobasal gradient in the distribution of these substances.

When cytological observations (page 42) brought evidence of an apicobasal gradient of basophilic substances in the cytoplasm, this led to the supposition that they might originate in the nucleoli, and be rich in ribosomes, thus reinforcing the hypothesis advanced by Hämmerling. Moreover, when the regeneration of the apex of nucleate fragments of *Acetabularia* was studied, it became evident that the former could be renewed within a few hours. In the course of this process, the apex becomes exceedingly rich in substances which stain with azure blue and acetic azocarmine. Nucleolar volume and staining capacity falls concurrently, though more rapidly; the smaller the size of the fragments, the more marked is this reduction in size. In some cases, the nucleolar mass rounds up, and loses its basophilia, whereas the perinuclear zone becomes filled with granules or dense masses which can be stained with the usual reagents (Puiseux-Dao, 1962, 1965). These findings seem to confirm the idea that the apex of the alga contains morphogenetic substances of nuclear origin.

The normal alga is characterised by distinct polarity; the rhizoid contains the nucleus and new whorls and, finally, caps are formed at the other end of the cylindrical siphon. This polarity is usually maintained in nucleate fragments and even in stalks deprived of nuclei. However, very occasionally, a reproductive cap may form at both ends of this type of fragment (Hämmerling, 1934, 1936). A few rather exceptional findings encountered in cultures of *Acetabularia mediterranea* (Hämmerling, 1953, 1955a,b) and also in *Batophora* (Puiseux-Dao, 1962) seem to indicate that the presence of the nucleus is decisive for the formation of the rhizoids. Indeed, when the daughter nuclei deriving from the large, trophic, dividing nucleus have reached the reproductive organ, if the cytoplasm is very abundant, enough cytoplasmic debris may remain in the stalk for germination to occur there: cytoplasmic zones containing a nucleus then secrete a membrane and grow within the stalk, or sometimes even in the cap; rhizoids develop near the nucleus. A similar phenomenon takes place when the cysts of a certain number of Dasycladales germinate directly to give rise to a new alga: a new algal thread grows out through the opening formed by the lid of the cysts which, at this stage, still contain a single nucleus, and are still lodged in the parent plant (Puiseux-Dao, 1962).

While the nucleus certainly influences the cytoplasm and cell morphology, the converse is equally true, as is indicated by the transformation of the nucleoli in differing culture conditions. Moreover, as early as in 1939, and once more in 1953, Hämmerling showed that nuclear division as well as nuclear morphology depended on the state of the cytoplasm. If the algal cap is removed just prior to division, the latter does not occur until a new reproductive organ has been elaborated: nuclear division may be retarded in this way for at least two years. The grafting of a still very young nuclear fragment on to an anucleate portion having a reproductive cap in an advanced stage of development causes nuclear division to occur about 15 days later, although under normal conditions it would be delayed for another two months at least. Moreover, the algae which contain a nucleus form their cap later than *Acetabularia* of the same age which have had their nucleus removed: the presence of the nucleus delays the morphogenesis of the reproductive organs (Beth, 1953b).

B. INTRA- AND INTERSPECIFIC GRAFTS

Remarkable interspecific grafts were first made in 1940, between various species of *Acetabularia*. If two freshly severed portions of *Acetabularia* are fitted into one another before the cuts have healed, the cytoplasm of the two portions unites at their meeting point and a huge cell, or 'transplantat', is formed, having two nuclei deriving from the same or different species according to the origin of the fragments (*Acetabularia mediterranea* and *crenulata*, for instance). This 'hybrid' alga grows and elaborates one or more reproductive organs. In the main, it looks like a reversed T, since its growth continues perpendicularly to the axis of the two grafts, from the point of junction. These algae are *fertile* when the graft is intraspecific and *sterile*, in most cases, when interspecific. In the latter case, the cap displays characteristics intermediary between those of the two species (Fig. 16); it is called 'Zwischenhut' (Hämmerling, 1940, 1943b).

This kind of experiment has not been restricted to nuclear fragments only; anucleate portions have also been grafted upon other fragments with or without a nucleus. Grafts totally lacking a nucleus which are able to grow have been achieved between *mediterranea* and *crenulata*. When the grafted fragments have been taken from flourishing algae are sufficiently large and, most important of all, if they are apical, they elaborate a sterile cap of intermediate form, closer in its morphological characteristics to *crenulata* than to *mediterranea*. In the case of graft containing one nucleus which generally becomes fertile, elongation occurs in the terminal part opposite to the nucleus, as in the normal algae; confirmation is thus provided of the existence of polarity depending on the presence of the nucleus. In interspecific grafts the cap formed bears a greater resemblance to the species which supplied the nucleus; traces of the character of the other alga are also displayed, however, especially in the case of apical fragments coming from *Acetabularia crenulata* and nucleate parts coming from *A. mediterranea*. If in such grafts the first cap formed is cut off, the graft elaborates another, the characteristics of which are a pure expression of the species which has furnished the nucleus. This again witnesses to the existence of Hämmerling's morphogenetic substances of nuclear origin. The substances stored in the axial stalk would explain, as we have seen, the capacity of the anucleate fragments to regenerate and to influence the form of the first cap in the latter case of a uninucleate graft. The slight domination of the species *crenulata* over the species

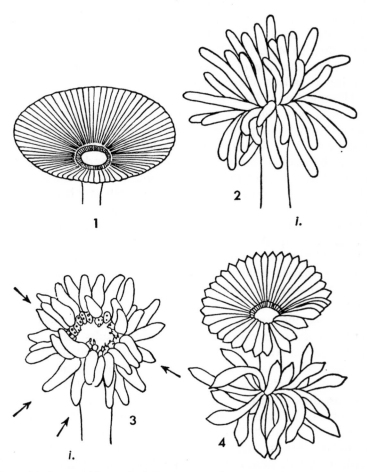

Figure 16. Interspecific grafts between *A. mediterranea* and *A. crenulata*. (1) Normal cap of *A. mediterranea* formed of 72 contiguous chambers (or rays), without spurs. (2) Intermediate cap (i) of *A. crenulata-mediterranea*. The composite heterozygote possesses a nucleus belonging to each species. The cap is made up of 33 distinctly separate chambers, without spurs. (3) Intermediate cap form (i) close to the species *crenulata* formed by a heterozygote containing two *cren*-nuclei and only one from *med*-. This cap has 34 rays, some of which are pointed (arrow). (4) Normal caps of *A. crenulata*. The rays (chambers), about 35 of which are present, are spurred and united to a variable extent. (After Hämmerling, 1953.)

mediterranea should be mentioned: the German authors concluded that a greater quantity of morphogenetic substances would be present in the former. However, qualitative, differences are involved. The rate of protein synthesis would, according to Werz (1957b) be higher in *crenulata*, which would determine the rate of protein synthesis in heterozygotes containing a nucleus of each type.

Hämmerling (1946b) produced trinucleate algae by amputating the new outgrowth from a graft containing two different nuclei, and by implanting it into a freshly prepared nuclear fragment. Werz (1955) studied all the possible combinations of grafts between *Acetabularia mediterranea* and *crenulata* from uninucleate to quadrinucleate combinations. Such experiments showed that the morphology of the generally sterile caps formed depends on the nuclei present; the more nuclei of any one species that are present, the more this species dominates at the level of the cap. A varying scale of diverse combinations is thus obtained among the resulting intergrades. Let us mention, in passing, that each nucleus in a plurinuclear specimen is inferior in size to what is thought of as normal for the given species (Werz, 1955).

Interspecific grafts, other than those uniting *mediterranea* and *crenulata*, have given very variable results. Beth (1943b,c) and Maschlanka (1943, 1964) obtained different sterile heterozygotes of *mediterranea—acicularia*. In the same way, after grafting, *Acetabularia mediterranea* and *Acetabularia peniculus* can produce hybrids bearing intermediate caps (Puiseux-Dao, unpublished; Plate 11). In both cases, however, the interspecific specimen is much less successful than with *mediterranea—crenulata*. Trials which were even less fruitful have been made with *Acetabularia wettsteinii* and *polyphysoides* grafted either on *mediterranea* or on *crenulata*. These rather unsuccessful attempts have inspired the thought that genetically, the two species are too widely separated to produce anything but rare monstrous caps. Also, uninucleate grafts developed by *mediterranea-wettsteinii* form caps characteristic of the species which supplies the nucleus; the anucleate portion has no effect, except for plastids and membranous remnants reminiscent of the species which did not give the nucleus (Hämmerling, 1934b, 1953).

The well-defined morphology of the caps elaborated by *Acetabularia mediterranea* and *crenulata* usefully permit a comparison of the degree of influence exerted by each of the nuclei present, and thus supply a means of checking the results obtained by other experimental techniques. For instance irradiated algae only form their caps with difficulty after receiving a certain threshold dose of X-ray irradiation; similarly, when algae so treated are grafted upon another species of *Acetabularia* which has not been irradiated, they have a lesser influence upon the form of the intermediate cap (Six and Puiseux-Dao, 1961).

C. IMPLANTATION OF NUCLEI INTO ANUCLEATE FRAGMENTS

Delicate methods for isolating nuclei have been developed in Germany (Hämmerling, 1955b; Richter, 1959b; Werz, 1962). The nucleate fragment, that is to say the algal base, is placed in buffer solution containing sucrose, at a temperature of 4°C. Then, using fine forceps, the fragment is gently squeezed until the nucleus is ejected into the sucrose solution. The maximum survival time of these nuclei, in the above medium, is only about three minutes. But they can be injected, while still living, using a micropipette, into anucleate basal fragments aged more than three weeks which have subnormal or arrested synthetic activity. After such an operation, growth and morphogenesis of the previously enucleate fragments begin again, and the adult algae which result are able to form normal and fertile reproductive organs. Their behaviour is identical to that of a uninucleate graft between an anucleate non-apical segment which has 'grown old' and a basal part having a nucleus (Richter, 1958b, 1959b). Immediately after the transfer of the isolated nucleus, its volume diminishes, but afterwards returns to normal (Zetsche, 1963b). A further interesting fact is that the implanted nucleus confers new vitality upon the previous anucleate fragment. If, after implantation, the operated algae are kept in the dark, then cut to produce a new anucleate and a nucleate part and retransferred to light, the former has regained a higher capacity for morphogenesis than the controls in which no implantation of a nucleus has been made. The nucleus is thus able to emit morphogenetic substances in the dark (Zetsche, 1962). This is in good agreement with the conclusions reached on the basis of observations concerning the nucleolus (page 80). Although the new cell constituted by this implantation technique is vitally alive and independent, there is a very definite line of demarcation between the old part of the stalk, which has a thick membrane and dark green plastids, and the new germling, which is thin walled and light green, because of the different colour of the plastids; these cells become fertile (Schweiger et al., 1969).

This type of experiment tends to prove that the results obtained with grafting experiments are a consequence of the influence of the nucleus, rather than of the cytoplasmic portion which has been grafted with it.

These techniques of grafting and nuclear implantation are certainly a very valuable instrument in the study of nucleocytoplasmic relations and of the relationship between the nucleus and the cytoplasmic organelles containing satellite DNA.

5

The biochemistry of *Acetabularia*

As we have seen, the well-defined morphology of the giant unicellular alga, *Acetabularia*, and the ease with which nucleate and anucleate fragments can be obtained, makes this biological material extremely useful for studies of nucleocytoplasmic relationships. The prolonged survival of anucleate fragments encourages the supposition that many metabolic pathways function independently of direct nuclear control. Analysis has effectively shown that the cytoplasm is relatively autonomous with regard to the nucleus (Brachet, 1957, 1958b, 1961; Hämmerling, 1957, 1958, 1963a,b; Hämmerling et al., 1958; Schweiger, 1969).

A. BIOCHEMICAL ANALYSES OF NUCLEO-CYTOPLASMIC INTERRELATIONS

Preliminary experiments were designed with the aim of discovering which metabolic pathways are most disturbed by enucleation.

1. Respiration and photosynthesis

(a) RESPIRATION

A Warburg apparatus can be used to measure in the dark the rate of respiration in *Acetabularia mediterranea*. In this respect, similar results are obtained when equal quantities of nucleate and anucleate fragments are compared over a period of four to five weeks. Beyond that period the nucleate fragments enter a period of rapid regeneration, and their respiratory rate consequently rises, whereas the growth of the anucleate fragments comes to a stop (Chantrenne-Van Halteren and Brachet, 1952;

Brachet et al., 1955). Thus, there does not seem to be any direct relation between respiration and the presence of the nucleus. At all events, an inhibitor like trypaflavin, which reduces the uptake of oxygen by *Acetabularia* after a few days treatment, inhibits the development of both kinds of fragment (Stich, 1951b).

(b) PHOTOSYNTHESIS

The photosynthetic activity of the alga, as estimated using sea water to which $NaHCO_3$ ($1.5 . 10^{-2}M$) has been added, and in an atmosphere enriched in CO_2 (5%) seems to be relatively independent of nuclear control, since it is still comparable to that of nucleate controls four weeks after enucleation. This has been confirmed by an ever increasing number of publications, and is evidence of the functional autonomy of the plastids of *Acetabularia* (see Chapter 6).

2. *Phosphorus metabolism*

Enucleation does not immediately alter the metabolism of phosphorus; in this respect the alga differs from Amoeba, for which a quite opposite result has been obtained (Brachet et al., 1955). The addition of radioactive phosphorus, ^{32}P, to the culture medium, results in considerable uptake of the tracer into the nucleoli, and into cytoplasmic granules thought by Stich (1951) to be of meta- and polyphosphate nature. This incorporation is related to photosynthesis, since it does not occur when the algae are kept in the dark (Stich and Hämmerling, 1953; Hämmerling and Stich, 1954, 1956a,b). Anucleate stalks and nucleate fragments resemble one another in this respect; three months after enucleation, the uptake of ^{32}P is even more striking in certain types of fragments. The ATP content similarly escapes nuclear control, at least during the initial period immediately consecutive to the cutting of the alga; in this respect, also, *Acetabularia* differs from Amoeba (Brachet et al., 1955). Analysis of the lipid bound, inorganic, acid-soluble and alkali-soluble phosphorus of the alga also directed Schweiger and Bremer (1960a) to the conclusion that the metabolism of these different forms of phosphorus remains independent of the nucleus for at least one month. The only fraction which is an exception to this rule involves the nucleotide pool for RNAs.

3. *Nitrogen metabolism and protein synthesis*

(a) GENERAL STUDY OF THE METABOLISM OF NITROGEN

Protein synthesis in nucleate and anucleate fragments is identical during an initial period of two to three weeks, according to Chantrenne et al. (1953), Vanderhaeghe (1954), Brachet et al., (1955) and Clauss and Werz (1961); during that period, their protein content increases threefold. At the end of that time, protein synthesis falls progressively in anucleate fragments (Werz and Hämmerling, 1959) while it continues actively in those containing a nucleus (Fig. 17). Clauss (1958) makes a distinction between the proteins of the cytoplasm, the synthesis of which continues for about twenty days in the absence of the nucleus, and those of the chloroplasts; the latter behave in the

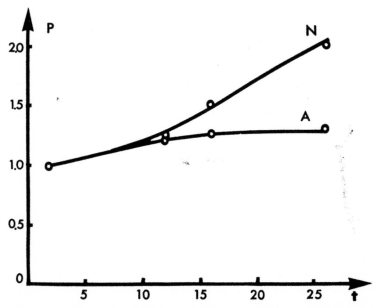

Figure 17. Evolution of protein nitrogen (P) (in μg of amino acid derived from the proteins of ten samples) as a function of time (t) in days after the severing of the nucleate (N) from the anucleate (A) fragment. (After Brachet et al., 1955.)

same way as the cytoplasmic proteins in the apical anucleate fragments, whereas in the basal parts protein synthesis stops from the seventh day onwards. This difference is probably due to the fact that the structure of the chloroplasts of the apex differs from those at the base of the stalk (Puiseux-Dao, 1962a, Boloukhère-Presburg, 1969). The chloroplasts in this zone contain large stores, and it has been found (Vanden Driessche and Bonotto, 1967) that the accumulation of fructosans in these organelles is quite definitely improved by enucleation, to the detriment of plastid membrane synthesis (Puiseux-Dao and Dazy, 1970; Puiseux-Dao, 1970).

The increase in the nitrogen content of non-protein substances is more rapid in anucleate than in nucleate fragments (Giardina, 1954), which is contrary to protein nitrogen. The two types of fragments indeed differ insofar as the evolution of acid-soluble nitrogen and protein nitrogen is concerned (Brachet et al., 1955). The content in soluble nitrogen is always higher in anucleate fragments, probably, according to these authors, because of an accumulation of amino acids. Bremer et al. (1962), analysing chromatograms of amino acids obtained from *Acetabularia* fragments with or without a nucleus, found that glutamic acid, aspartic acid, alanine and glycine are the most abundant amino acids; asparagine is also found in quite large quantities. According to these authors, the amino acid content of both nucleate and anucleate fragments remains the same over a period of about twenty days. Bremer and Schweiger (1960) have, on the other hand, brought evidence demonstrating an accumulation of NH_4^+ ions in the fragments deprived of a nucleus.

The essential fact remains that for a certain, quite prolonged period, synthesis continues in anucleate *Acetabularia*, then it diminishes little by little, and finally ceases completely. Some controversy still exists as to the possible accumulation of precursors, either amino acids or NH_4^+ ions. Thus, protein synthesis does not seem to be affected immediately by enucleation; it is nevertheless more sensitive, in the long run, to the absence of the nucleus than the other metabolic pathways we have already discussed, and it has also been studied with much greater precision.

(b) STUDY OF PROTEIN SYNTHESIS

Two methods have been used for this analysis: one being the

study of the incorporation of precursors into total proteins, the other involving the determination of the specific activity of certain enzymes in the nucleate and anucleate fragments.

(i) The incorporation into the proteins of nucleate and anucleate fragments of $^{14}CO_2$ ($HNa^{14}O_3$) or of glycine (C^{14}-glycine) is identical for about *two weeks* (Brachet and Chantrenne, 1951, 1952; Brachet and Brygier, 1953; Brachet et al., 1955); this is very good proof of the fact that during this time protein synthesis occurs in the absence of the nucleus. It should be mentioned that whatever the fragment studied, the incorporation of ^{14}C coming from $Na^{14}CO_3$ obviously depends upon photosynthesis and decreases in the dark; it is at least two or three times higher in the chloroplasts as compared with the microsomal fraction. The opposite is true for ^{14}C from glycine, which is incorporated to a much greater extent (50 to 100% more) into the microsomes than into the plastids, a phenomenon which does not depend on light conditions at all, since it takes place just as well in the dark as in the light. These authors came to the conclusion that protein synthesis in *Acetabularia* makes use not only of carbon chains elaborated during photosynthesis, but also of external supplies. Different strains of *Acetabularia*, and also *Batophora*, grow in a flourishing manner in sea water to which amino acids or amides have been added. The algae which, under such growth conditions, are intensely green, are able to carry on photosynthesis, but they nevertheless readily incorporate molecules offered by the external medium; the aminoacids which have been found to be most abundant on quantitative analysis (Bremer et al., 1962), in *Acetabularia* have also been found to be most favourable to growth (Puiseux-Dao, 1962a).

(ii) In order to check whether the synthesis of all these proteins is equally influenced by enucleation, the enzyme content of nucleate and anucleate fragments has been compared. Baltus (1959) has shown that aldolase activity persists in the absence of the nucleus and that the synthesis of this enzyme is still very marked after ten days. A similar result was obtained by Clauss (1959), who measured the activity of algal extracts with regard to solutions of glucose-1-phosphate: at the end of three weeks, the phosphorylase content stopped increasing. These two diastases are not localised in a cell organelle, but are almost ubiquitous within the algae, except perhaps in the microsomes in the case of aldolase. Invertase was also shown to be synthesised for some time after enucleation by Keck and Clauss (1959), who studied the activity of this enzyme, using saccharose as a substrate. The enzymes required for carbohydrate metabolism are not the only ones which seem to be synthesised in the anucleate fragments of *Acetabularia*; enzymes of other pathways may also be synthesised, for instance the ribonucleases which have been shown by Schweiger (1966) to exist in *Acetabularia*. Conversely, the synthesis of acid phosphatase, an enzyme tested on β-glycerophosphate, seemed at first to be quite impossible in the absence of the nucleus (Keck and Clauss, 1958; Vanderhaeghe-Hougardy and Baltus, 1962). But in fact, five distinct isoenzymes have been found to exist (Spencer and Harris, 1964; Triplett et al., 1965), three of which are found in sufficient quantity to be estimated. The activity of at least two of them has been found to increase readily in the absence of the nucleus; they are associated with the chloroplast fraction, and seem to be particularly active at the time of formation of the caps. A third isoenzyme, which is not bound to the plastids, gradually decreases in activity, in the course of time, in the anucleate fraction (Fig. 18).

These results lead to the general conclusion that a high proportion of the proteins of the cell can be elaborated by the anucleate cytoplasm even when their synthesis is known to be under nuclear control as has been shown for lactic deshydrogenase by Reuter and Schweiger (1969) and for malic deshydrogenase by Schweiger et al. (1969). In one case, protein synthesis has even been found to be more active in the anucleate than in the nucleate fragments, that is to say, in the amputated tips of *Acetabularia* removed just before the initiation of the reproductive cap (Brachet et al., 1955). The morphogenesis of the reproductive organs is naturally accompanied by intense metabolic activity located at the tip, where substances which probably originate in the nucleus accumulate in abundance, in greater quantity than at the base of the growing stalk (Werz, 1960a,b). Although the nucleate rhizoid fragments are capable of regenerating very rapidly and of producing a new apex, after a period of intense nucleolar emission (Puiseux-Dao, 1965), they certainly do not possess a higher concentration of these

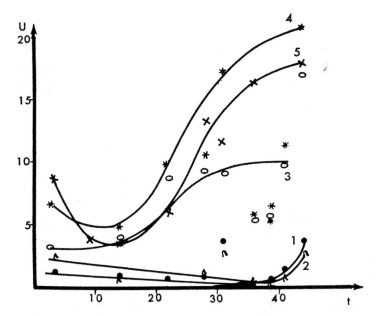

Figure 18. Evolution of the content in three isoenzymes of the acid phosphatase in *A. mediterranea* (anucleate parts). Differences in electrophoretic mobility make it possible to distinguish between the three isozymes; they are respectively: 1·04 (1); 3·12 (2); and 6·25 (3). The graphs numbered 4 and 5 give the total enzyme activity measured by a densitometric technique (4) or by the method of Fiske-Subbarow (5). *Abcissa*: time in days. *Ordinate*: enzyme activity in units per γ of protein-tyrosine. (After Triplett et al., 1965.)

substances than the normal stalk, and this could in fact explain the differences between the two isolated halves. Clauss (1962b) however seems to prove that there is but little increase in protein synthesis at the time of cap formation, and this is in good agreement with the findings of Shephard (1965a) and of Terborgh and Thimann (1965). The increase in weight due to the accumulation of proteins in the developing reproductive organ is merely the result of cytoplasmic movement within the stalk, terminating by its concentration within the cap; such upward cytoplasmic movements have been observed very clearly in several species (Schulze, 1939; Puiseux-Dao, 1962). Brachet and his collaborators have drawn a parallel between their results showing that the apical anucleate parts of *Acetabularia* are able to form a cap and are more active in protein synthesis than nucleate controls, and those of Beth (1953b) showing that the presence of the nucleus inhibits the formation of caps, perhaps because of competition for precursors. Furthermore, Stich and Kitiyara (1957) believe that inhibition by the cytoplasm of protein synthesis may exist, and may be lifted by the amputation of the algal stalk; Clauss (1962a) does not agree with this finding.

While it is unquestionable that protein synthesis can take place in the absence of the nucleus, it does not persist for more than three weeks in the anucleate algae, even under the best possible conditions. In comparison with other metabolic pathways, such as that of phosphorus, for instance, which remains functional two months after enucleation, it may be inferred that protein synthesis and nuclear metabolism bear some relationship to one another. Very affirmative confirmation of this relationship derives from experiments made by Richter (1959b): by grafting a part of a nucleate stalk or by injecting an isolated nucleus into an anucleate fragment more than three weeks old, it is possible to stimulate the renewal of active protein synthesis in cytoplasm in which such anabolism was previously completely arrested.

Since Brachet and Casperson ascribed to ribonucleic acids the role of intermediate between the nucleus and cytoplasmic protein synthesis as early as 1941, a great deal of experimental work has naturally aimed at investigating their behaviour.

4. The metabolism of RNAs
(Brachet, 1962b, 1963a, 1964, 1965a,b,c, 1968a,b)

Direct estimation soon showed that *Acetabularia mediterranea* contains net quantities of RNAs (Brachet et al., 1955). With cytochemical techniques, their presence can be detected in the nucleoli, in nucleolar emissions and at the tip of the stalks: the RNAs so detected are probably ribosomal, since other types of RNAs do not readily resist the usual cytochemical techniques (page 40).

The possibility that RNAs might be synthesised in anucleate fragments remained for a long time a subject of controversy. While it was rapidly established by many authors that removal

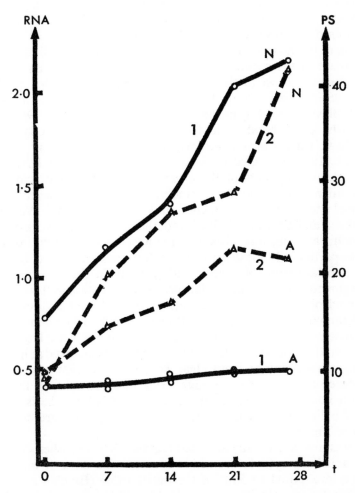

Figure 19. Evolution of the RNA content (1) and of the amount of soluble proteins (2) in the nucleate (N) and the anucleate (A) portions of *A. mediterranea*. *Abcissa*: time in days after cutting of the fragments. *Ordinate*: content in μg per sample. (After Richter, 1959a.)

of the nucleus influences RNA metabolism very considerably, some were more categorical than others and even denied any anabolic activity to the cytoplasmic RNAs after enucleation. It became quite clear that very refined techniques would be required to resolve this problem. Determination of RNA content by the technique of Ogur and Rosen failed to detect any increase in the amount of these nucleic acids in the anucleate fragments grown in the usual way; these findings led to the conclusion that no synthesis of RNAs takes place in the cytoplasm lacking a nucleus (Fig. 19) (Richter, 1957, 1959a,b). On the other hand, right from the beginning methods using isotopic tracers have always (with only one exception—Naora et al., 1959) provided evidence of the anabolism of RNAs in anucleate fragments of the algae. Indeed, ^{14}C-orotic acid and ^{14}C-adenine were found to be incorporated by both nucleate and anucleate fragments (Brachet and Szarfarz, 1953; Vander-haeghe and Szarfarz, 1955; Vanderhaeghe, 1957; Naora et al., 1960); labelling was weaker in the absence of the nucleus and was particularly localised in the chloroplast fraction (Fig. 20). A constant ratio of specific radioactivity in the two types of fragments was recorded. Measurement of the content of RNA bound phosphorus (method derived from that of Schmidt and Thannhauser, Schweiger and Bremer, 1960b, 1961) showed an increase in the total quantity of cytoplasmic RNAs. However, it should be mentioned that these experiments involved anucleate fragments obtained from algae kept in the dark for ten days before sectioning, then brought back into the light. In fact, in both nucleate and anucleate fragments, RNA synthesis drops in the dark, and recommences when the fragments are brought back into the light.

It is now a generally accepted fact that RNA synthesis occurs in anucleate cytoplasm; within four to nine days. it may rise to a level equal to 50% of the initial value (Brachet and Six, 1966). Frequently, it may even double within one week (Brachet, 1968b). Nevertheless, the absence of the nucleus indubitably alters the metabolism of ribonucleic acids, and for this reason it became important to discover which of the cytoplasmic RNAs is most sensitive to enucleation.

Although technical difficulties (including the presence in *Acetabularia* of very active ribonucleases which are not easily inhibited) made this task difficult, Janowsky undertook investigations (1963, 1965) tending to discover which types of RNA would be synthesised after enucleation. The RNAs extracted from algae labelled with ^{32}P were fractionated by column chromatography on methylated albumin, and three kinds of RNA were found to become radioactive in the absence of the nucleus.

(i) An RNA of low molecular weight which is either transfer RNA or a degradation product of bigger molecules which are found everywhere in the cytoplasm.

(ii) RNA of ribosomal type localised in the plastids.

(iii) Another type of chloroplastid RNA closely associated with the DNA of these organelles, described by Richter (1966b) and which may correspond to the rapidly labelled RNA present in whole algae and in the anucleate stalk.

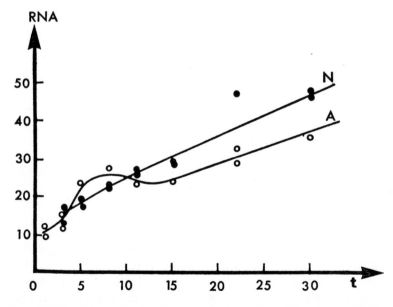

Figure 20. Evolution of the RNA content in the nucleate (N) and the anucleate (A) fragments of *A. mediterranea*. *Abcissa*: time in days after amputation. *Ordinate*: average RNA content of one fragment (in 10^{-5} μM). (After Brachet et al., 1955.)

The isolated plastids are also able to incorporate precursors into 23, 16, 9 and 4S RNAs (Berger, 1967); this incorporation is inhibited by lack of light, deoxyribonuclease and actinomycin.

In fact, RNAs are synthesised in the plastids, the mitochondria and in the hyaloplasm (supernatant), not only by nucleate, but also by anucleate fragments. ^{14}C-uracil is effectively incorporated into RNAs from these different fractions and when separated in sucrose gradients after labelling of the algae for six days, the curves obtained resemble those obtained with ribosomal RNA from *Escherischia coli* (Schweiger et al., 1967). The degree of labelling of nucleate and anucleate fragments or whole algae with radioactive precursors is found to be very comparable (Dillard, 1970; Dillard and Schweiger, 1968a,b), a finding which causes little surprise when it is remembered that the plastids taken all together contain 1,000 to 10,000 times more DNA than the nucleus.

A general investigation of cytoplasmic ribosomes and polysomes was made by Janowski (1966, 1967), Janowski et al. (1968) and by Baltus et al. (1968). In these experiments whole algae or fragments of such were labelled with ^{3}H-uridine (100 μc/ml for two hours) or with a mixture of ^{14}C-amino acids. The radioactivity present in extracted fractions was studied by sucrose gradient analysis before and after treatment with dilute ribonuclease, used at a concentration destined to destroy the messenger RNAs which link the ribosomes together to form polysomes. In normal *Acetabularia*, radioactivity after incorporation of ^{3}H-uridine is especially found in three peaks having sedimentation coefficients of 70, 50 and 30 (Fig. 21); the 50S particles seem to contain labelled 23S RNAs, whereas the 30S particles contain radioactivity due to 16S RNAs. After treatment with ribonuclease, the '70' peak increases in height, finding which may be interpreted as due to the conversion of the polysomes to 70S monomers. If the concentration of Mg^{2+} ions in the homogenising medium is increased, the only result is a diminished yield of polysomes, and it is therefore very unlikely that the 50 and 30S components are subunits of monosomes. Two days after cutting the algae, the anucleate halves are still able to incorporate uridine into the polysomes, the 70, 50 and 30S particles, but a comparatively lower transfer of the radioactivity of the polysomes to 70S ribosomes occurs after treat-

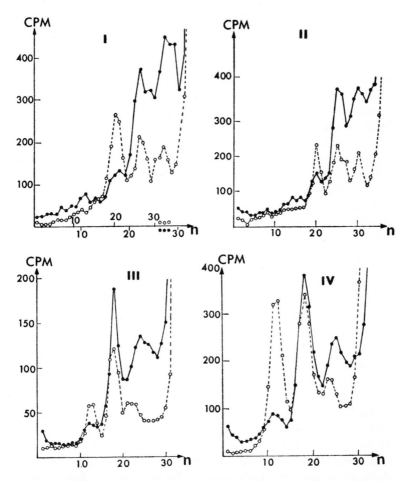

Figure 21. Sedimentation profile of cytoplasmic ribosomes of *A. mediterranea* labelled with ³H-uridine. The algae were placed for 2 hrs in the usual culture medium containing ³H-uridine (100 μc/ml). The centrifugation was carried out in a sucrose gradient (15 to 30%; 4·8 ml) for 2 hrs at a speed of 37,000 rpm (Spinco 450 centrifuge, rotor SW 39). Normal samples (continuous); samples treated with ribonuclease (broken line). (I) Whole plants: the final concentration of Mg++ in the homogenate = 5·10⁻³ M. (II) Whole plants: the concentration of Mg++ in the homogenate = 8·10⁻³ M. (III) Two-day anucleate fragments that were allowed to regenerate in the light. (IV) Two-day anucleate fragments that were allowed to regenerate in the dark. (After Brachet, 1968.)

ment with ribonuclease. On the other hand, when anucleate fragments are maintained in obscurity prior to experimentation, labelling of all the RNA fractions, including the polysomes, is greatly increased; moreover, after treatment with ribonuclease, the 70S peak markedly augments. These results concur with the assays made on whole algae by Schweiger and Bremer (1961) and tend to suggest that polysomes are elaborated in the absence of the nucleus in *Acetabularia*. The strong influence of light on the labelling of anucleate fragments raises the question of a possible synthesis of messenger RNAs for these active polysomes on plastid DNA, irrespective of their site of action as informational macromolecules which may, or may not, be outside the plastids (Brachet, 1968).

Janowski et al. (1969) undertook to estimate and to localise the different categories of ribosomes and ribosomal subunits in cell fractions. Whereas only negative results were obtained for the hyaloplasm, chloroplasts were effectively found to contain 70, 50 and 30S particles, and ribosomal synthesis actually persists in these organelles for four weeks after enucleation in complete agreement with the observations made by Naora et al. (1960). Although chloramphenicol inhibits the incorporation of uridine into the RNA of the polysomes and of the 70S particles, it only irregularly affects the synthesis of the 50S and 30S particles; once again, this finding suggests there is no relationship between 70S particles and those sedimenting at 50S and 30S.

As for the ribosomal RNAs themselves, Baltus and Quertier (1966) have isolated the 16S and 25S RNAs of the *Acetabularia*; at least one of these, perhaps even both, disappear in the anucleate algae (Dillard and Schweiger, 1968a,b) although there is no apparent reduction in the number of ribosomes. In particular, particles of a ribosomal type can be observed in these fragments; one can only speculate on their content in RNAs (Baltus et al., 1968; Janowski and Bonotto, in Brachet, 1968; Dillard and Schweiger, 1968).

Using an appropriate extraction technique, involving precipitation of high molecular weight nucleic acids with a two molar solution of lithium chloride, followed by extraction with phenol, Farber (in Brachet, 1968) managed to isolate three large RNAs (I, II and III) from whole *Acetabularia* and from fragments deprived of a nucleus. Fraction I seems to disappear at the time of formation of the reproductive cap, whereas fraction III is rapidly labelled with uridine during 'pulse' experiments. The disappearance of fraction I seems to coincide with a decrease in the ability to incorporate radioactive amino acids in an appropriate *in vitro* system, stimulated by total RNA (Farber et al., 1969).

A study of the base composition of the RNAs localised in different parts of the algae should bring further elements of understanding to this field. Microelectrophoretic techniques have for instance so far furnished the following data (Baltus et al., 1968).

(i) The RNA of the nucleolus is complementary to nuclear DNA in that a close correlation between the proportions of A and U and G and C is observed; the adenine (A) content of the nucleolus is also very similar to that of the DNA of the gametes. This exceptional base composition of the nucleolar RNA of *Acetabularia* can be compared with that of the same organelle in the salivary glands of *Chironomus*, which similarly shows non-conformity to the general rule of high guanine content for nucleolar RNA.

(ii) The base composition of the nucleoplasmic RNAs differs from that of the nucleolar RNAs. They are particularly rich in uridine (U), in agreement with observations made on other biological materials.

(iii) The ribosomes of the plastids are rich in GC; when the total RNA of the plastids is compared to the pool of ribosomal RNAs, the GC percentages are observed to differ, implying the presence of RNAs other than ribosomal.

(iv) There is no apparent difference between the RNAs isolated from the tip of the alga and those obtained from its base; this apparent homogeneity might, however, be due to cyclotic movements.

As can be seen, the study of RNAs of *Acetabularia* is a complicated problem, which can only be investigated in three different systems at present: either the whole algae, or anucleate fragments, or, again, isolated plastids. The latter are quite autonomous organelles from this point of view, possessing their own DNA, ribosomal particles defined as 70, 50 and 30S, their own ribosomal type RNA rich in GC forming the 23 and 16S RNAs which contains a stable component, as well as the 9S and 4S RNAs. The mitochondria are undoubtedly similarly equipped. Less complete information is available as far as the nucleus and the hyaloplasm is concerned. The nucleoplasm quite classically, contains RNAs which are rich in uridine, whereas the nucleolus would seem to contain a higher concentration of DNA like RNAs than is usually the case. The nucleolus plays a role in the production of cytoplasmic and perhaps chloroplastic ribosomes, and its loss would be the reason for the fall in content of ribosomal RNAs observed in anucleate fragments. This apparent disappearance of ribosomal RNAs might however result from the operational shock consecutive to cutting (Dillard, 1970) or to an arrest of the autonomous ribosomal synthesis in plastids (Puiseux-Dao, 1970). Possible relationships between 70, 50 and 30S ribosomal particles and the ribosomes themselves, have yet to be elucidated. Also the high molecular weight RNAs have not yet been satisfactorily identified. The technical problems raised by biochemical estimations soon promoted diverse laboratories to elaborate different methods of study; autoradiography is certainly one of the most fruitful.

B. AUTORADIOGRAPHIC ANALYSIS OF NUCLEOCYTOPLASMIC INTERRELATIONS

Given the preliminary results obtained by biochemical methods, autoradiography was obviously primarily concerned with the precursors of nucleic acids and of proteins. Experiments were generally planned in the following way: on the one hand, labelling experiments were carried out on normal algae, nucleate fragments undergoing regeneration, and anucleate segments fixed after having been kept for a given period in a radioactive medium; on the other hand, 'chase' experiments were undertaken by fixing the same materials after an initial period in radioactive medium, followed by a 'chase' in the same medium lacking the radioactive precursor. In both types of experiment, algae cultured in light, or in the dark, were compared.

1. The normal metabolism of RNAs in Acetabularia mediterranea

The first autoradiographic experiments concerning the metabolism of RNAs were carried out with ^{32}P phosphorus in the form of PO_4^{3-} (Stich and Hämmerling, 1953 and Hämmerling and Stich, 1956a,b), then with ^{14}C-orotic acid and ^{14}C-adenine (Vanderhaeghe, 1957). As methods of synthesis of radioactive precursors improved, Werz and Zetsche (1962) were able to work with ^{14}C-uracil, while de Vitry employed 5-methyl-cytosine (1963), then tritium-labelled uridine, cytidine and guanosine (1965a,b,c); the use of the latter is, however, limited by its relative toxicity. The technique of fixation by freeze substitution seems to be particularly suitable for this research, the specificity of labelling is usually controlled in one or several ways. Treatments with perchloric acid (2%, 5°C, 20 minutes), which removes the nucleotides and the free peptides, or with normal hydrochloric acid (60°C, 5 minutes) which eliminates the RNAs and the purine bases of DNA were very useful. Enzyme digestions with ribonuclease (0·2 mg/ml for $1\frac{1}{2}$ hours at 37°C) or with deoxyribonuclease (0·2 mg/ml for $1\frac{1}{2}$ hours at 37°C) were also convenient. The sections so treated were of course compared with controls (de Vitry, 1965a).

Whatever the precursor used, the results obtained corroborate the following findings (de Vitry, 1965a). Under normal culture conditions, in the light, nuclear incorporation— particularly into the nucleolus, dominates during the first three hours. Subsequently, cytoplasmic radioactivity increases progressively with time, while, after twenty-four hours, nuclear labelling reaches a plateau or may even drop (Fig. 22). At the end of one day, the distribution of silver grains in the autoradiographic emulsion signalises the existence of a definite apico basal gradient, with high apical density, which is steadily attenuated along the length of the stalk, up to the perinuclear zone which is also characterised by intense labelling. When the algae are maintained in darkness during this experiment, no gradient occurs: labelling is dense in the nucleus and in the surrounding cytoplasm, but remains low in the algal stalk.

Chase experiments, carried out with illuminated *Acetabularia* kept in a radioactive medium for twenty-four hours, demonstrate a gradual decrease in nuclear radioactivity accom-

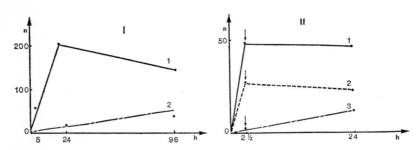

Figure 22. Autoradiographic study of the metabolism of RNAs in *A. mediter-ranea*. (I) Incorporation of ^{3}H-uridine into the nucleoli (1) and into the cytoplasm (2). (II) Evolution of labelling (2 h 30) with ^{3}H-uridine followed by a chase, in the nucleoli (1), in the nucleoplasm (2) and in the apical cytoplasm (3). *Abcissa*: time (t) in hrs. *Ordinate*: number of traces per 100 μ^2. (After de Vitry, 1965.)

panied by a rise in cytoplasmic labelling (de Vitry, 1965a).

Studies of the evolution of labelling when the algae are placed for only two hours thirty minutes (pulse labelling) in the presence of a radioactive precursor before being returned to 'cold' sea water bring evidence of initial radioactivity in the nucleus only, diminishing during the 'chase' more quickly in the nucleoplasm than in the nucleolus. Labelling disappears only slowly, and is only lost in a significant manner after four days' chase. At the same time, it increases little by little in the cyto-plasm (Fig. 22). The apico-basal gradient appears in the stalk if the algae are kept in the light, but not if they are kept in the dark.

The nucleate fragments (de Vitry, 1965a) involving the lower third of the plants show exactly the same pattern of labelling as the whole algae. As for the anucleate stalks (de Vitry, 1965), their radioactivity increases slowly in the course of time, and is uniformly distributed; it becomes much weaker in the dark (Figs. 23 and 24). Labelling is always relatively lower than in nucleate fragments, except in the case of 5-methyl cytosine, which produces exceptionally high labelling in the anucleate fragments (de Vitry, 1963).

These results show that the earliest site of RNA synthesis in the alga is the nucleus, the nucleolus being a particularly active site of synthesis or reorganisation. A small proportion of the RNAs produced by the nucleus (-15%) as calculated by

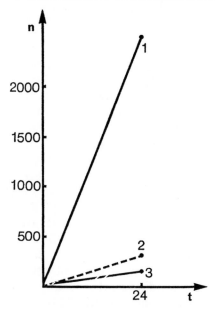

Figure 23. Incorporation of ^{3}H-cytidine into the nucleate and anucleate fragments of *A. mediterranea*. (1) Nucleoli. (2) Anucleate cytoplasm. (3) Nucleate cytoplasm. (After de Vitry, 1965.)

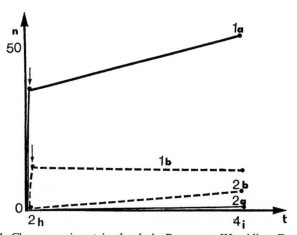

Figure 24. Chase experiment in the dark. Precursor: ^{3}H-uridine. Duration o labelling in the light = 2 hours (arrow). Only the radioactivity which could be eliminated by ribonuclease was taken into consideration. (1) Nucleoli. (2) Cytoplasm: (a) whole algae; (b) nucleate fragments. *Abcissa*: time (t). *Ordinate*: number of tracks per 100 μ^2 (n). (After de Vitry, 1965.)

quantitative studies of radioactive traces after chase experiments, move into the cytoplasm (+40%). The distribution of these RNAs corresponds exactly to the gradient established by Hämmerling for the morphogenetic substances of nuclear origin which control the morphogenesis of the algae (page 54). Ribonucleic acids are certainly among the morphogenetic substances produced by the nucleus and they probably include messengers manufactured in the nucleoplasm on DNA templates. Most of the RNAs of nuclear origin in Eucaryotes are ribosomal, however, their precursors being elaborated in the nucleolus by a relatively slow process (Attardi et al., 1967; Scherrer et al., 1967). Moreover, the anucleate cytoplasm is able to manufacture a certain amount of RNAs and, indubitably, the plastids and the mitochondria are at least in part responsible for this synthesis (page 111). The loss of the gradient in cytoplasmic labelling when the algae are deprived of light permits the supposition that if the synthesis of nuclear RNAs persists under such conditions, their transport from the base to the tip of the alga is suppressed. This transfer is certainly related to the cyclotic movements which require ATP, the main source of which in this biological material, is photosynthesis. The results obtained with 5-methyl cytosine remain difficult to explain. Moreover, it should be remembered that ^{32}P is incorporated at relatively high speed in the cytoplasm, in the presence of light only, at the level of granules which Stich (1953) identifies as meta- or polyphosphates. The presence of polyphosphates in *Acetabularia* has effectively been demonstrated (Thilo et al., 1965; Brachet and Lievens, in press).

2. *The normal metabolism of proteins in Acetabularia mediterranea*

Concurrently, protein anabolism has been investigated. The amino acids which have been used include: methionine (Olszewska and Brachet, 1960, 1961; Olszewska, de Vitry and Brachet, 1961), phenylalanine, tryptophan, arginine and lysine (de Vitry, 1965d) and serine (Werz and Zetsche, 1963). These amino acids fall into two categories: firstly, those which are instantaneously incorporated into the nucleus and the nucleate and anucleate cytoplasm, producing a degree of labelling which ncreases progressively in the course of time, and secondly, protein precursors whose incorporation kinetics run parallel to those of RNA precursors. Tryptophan, phenylalanine and arginine, present everywhere in these algae, fall into the first group, whereas methionine, serine and lysine belong to the second group. For instance, the nucleoli incorporate ten times more methionine than the surrounding cytoplasm during the first hour of incubation. When, after pulse labelling for one hour, the algae are replaced in a medium containing cold methionine, nuclear radioactivity drops little by little, whereas that of the cytoplasm increases; similarly, the tip of the algae is preponderantly labelled (Fig. 25). This confirms the occurrence of protein synthesis everywhere in the cell and tends, further, to suggest that basic proteins (cf. lysine) and proteins rich in sulphur accompany the RNAs of nuclear origin in their migration towards the apical zone of morphogenesis; these substances constitute, at least in part, the 'morphogenetic substances'.

Serine can be incorporated into RNA and for this reason, labelling with this amino acid is less significant than the others; however, when nuclear fragments labelled with ^{14}C-serine were

T	1	3	7	1	3	7
3 mm	1·33	3·05	3·41	1·25	6·16	5·77
	1·13	1·33	2·47	0·75	3·13	2·94
3 mm	0·30	1·11	2·36	0·38	2·11	1·86
6 mm						
5 mm	0·27	0·72	1·75	0·94	1·88	4·58
	0·27	0·50	1·41	0·69	1·11	3·58
3 mm	0·25	0·27	0·55	0·52	0·47	1·22
	3·66	3·88	3·62	2·86	9·44	8·91

Figure 25. Incorporation of ^{35}S-dl-methionine as a function of time in days, expressed as number of tracks per 100 μ^2 in different regions of the alga *A. mediterranea*. (After Olszewska and Brachet, 1961.)

grafted on to normal anucleate fragments, Werz and Zetsche (1963) observed that the apex became radioactive in the course of experimentation, thus bringing clear evidence in support of the nuclear origin of the apical substances newly formed in the uninucleate grafts.

Succinctly, on the basis of these findings the following conclusions may be drawn.

(i) RNA synthesis mainly occurs in the nucleus, both nucleolus and nucleoplasm playing an active role in this respect. But it must be borne in mind that biochemical results tend to imply a more important role for cytoplasm.

(ii) Some of the cytoplasmic RNAs are synthesised in the cytoplasm, but many of them are elaborated in the nucleus and are usually distributed along an apicobasal gradient. This gradient is nonexistent in algae kept in the dark, transport of substances of nuclear origin into the cytoplasm being slowed down under these circumstances.

(iii) Certain nuclear, probably messenger and ribosomal, RNAs migrate towards the apex of the alga together with basic proteins and proteins rich in sulphur; they may well correspond to morphogenetic substances.

(iv) Nucleus and cytoplasm are partially independent sites of protein synthesis.

C. THE EFFECTS OF INHIBITORS ON THE PATHWAY: DNA-RNAs-PROTEINS

Primarily, morphological effects produced by inhibitors were studied. Attempts were made to analyse the anomalies resulting from such treatments, using cytological and biochemical methods. Autoradiography was the most frequently used technique.

1. The effects of radiations

X-rays and ultraviolet rays were at first used to inhibit *Acetabularia* metabolism; gamma radiations are now also employed. Of course, such radiations only exert a visible effect above a certain threshold dose, and excessive doses are inevitably lethal.

(a) X-RAYS

Irradiation of the entire alga with 6 kiloroentgen causes cytoplasmic lesions, at least in the apical zone, from the twentieth day onwards. The stronger the irradiation, the more extensive are the lesions and the sooner they appear (after two days at 240 kiloroentgens and 720 kiloroentgens, for instance). In general, *Acetabularia* are able to regenerate after irradiation, and grow even more quickly than the controls. After very high doses, however, the plants become abnormal; morphogenesis is disturbed, but the algae survive. After an irradiation level of 750 kiloroentgens, the rhizoids themselves die and can no longer grow and regenerate (Bacq et al., 1957, Fig. 26).

If the rhizoids alone are irradiated, the stalks being given protection by lead, lesions are observed in the cytoplasm after twenty days with doses of 24 kiloroentgens and 72 kiloroentgens, and after two days with higher doses. Regeneration occurred in

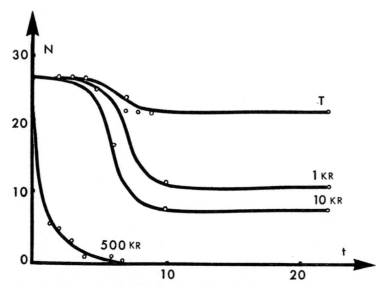

Figure 26. Survival of *A. mediterranea* irradiated *in toto* by X-rays as a function of time (t) in days. (T) controls; (N) number of stalks which survive; (KR) kiloroentgen. (After Bacq et al., 1957.)

all the samples from the rhizoids and the caps formed cysts (Bacq et al., 1957). When nucleate fragments of *Acetabularia* are irradiated for one to two days after cutting, the algae which develop are normal if the irradiations are below 200 kiloroentgens. The higher the dose, the greater is the reduction of growth rate. Above 400 kiloroentgens, some of the irradiated algae underwent cytoplasmic contractions and usually died. Their regenerative capacity diminished in proportion to the dose, the number of caps which could be elaborated followed the same law, and so did the formation and the fertility of the cysts in the reproductive organs. The duration of life of irradiated anucleate fragments, more sensitive than nucleate parts, depends on the dose received. Survival is definitely limited after doses of 200 and 300 kiloroentgens, and may be completely nil after doses of 400 kiloroentgens or more, according to the experiments; the possibility of growth and morphogenesis, especially of the cap, is reduced in the same way, in proportion to the dose (Fig. 27) (Hämmerling, 1956; Six, 1956b, 1958). In some experimental series, however, regeneration of nucleate and anucleate fragments was only slightly slowed down, or even a little accelerated for irradiations of 10 to 100 kiloroentgens; with 500 kiloroentgens, however, the deleterious effects observed by the German authors were found (Bacq et al., 1957).

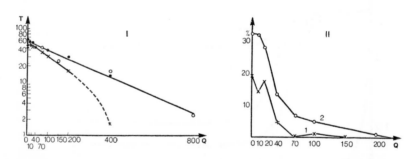

Figure 27. X-rays. (I) Average time of survival (T) in days of anucleate apical fragments of *A. mediterranea* as a function of the daily dose of irradiation, Q, in kiloroentgens, in several experimental series. (○) series 1; (●) average of series 1 and 2; (X) average of two other series. (II) Morphogenetic capacity of the cap (in %) of the anucleate apical fragments of *A. mediterranea* irradiated, as a function of the dose, Q, of irradiation in kiloroentgens. (1) Percentage of caps having a diameter of 1·2 mm or more. (2) Total percentage of caps and rudiments of caps. (After Six, 1956b.)

Interspecific grafts (*mediterranea—crenulata*) between plants which are irradiated and others which have not been irradiated show that above a certain dose, the nucleus of the irradiated alga loses its influence on the morphology of the intermediate cap which is formed (Six and Puiseux-Dao, 1961).

It emerges from these results that the cytoplasm seems to be more sensitive to X-rays than the nucleus which is, it is true, protected by a thick membrane. The anucleate fragments are more susceptible to damage. Moreover, morphogenesis has been found to be more sensitive to radiation damage than the simple survival of the algae.

(b) ULTRAVIOLET RAYS

Just as for X-rays, the survival of the algae has been studied, as well as their morphogenetic capacity. Cytoplasmic lesions which are more or less extensive, and which disappear after the regeneration of the nucleate part (which remains normal) are the most constantly observed effects. The stalk, as was the case with X-rays, is more sensitive than the rhizoids. Irradiation of the cytoplasm alone is almost as deleterious as irradiation of the entire alga. On the other hand, if the nucleate part alone is irradiated, the effect upon the alga is practically nil; in some cases there was even an activation of growth and morphogenesis (Errera and Vanderhaeghe, 1957).

The nucleate fragments are but little affected by ultraviolet rays, except when strong lethal doses are employed. In fact, except in the presence of lethal doses, the algae always undergo normal regeneration; the caps form fertile cysts. On the other hand, the anucleate stalk is much more easily damaged by uv: survival time and morphogenetic capacity are both strongly reduced. Six (1956a, 1958) was able to demonstrate the variability in radiation effect, according to the wavelength. The wavelength of 254 millimicrons is the most dangerous; that of 281 millimicrons is a little less, while 297 millimicrons have almost no effect on the nucleate and anucleate fragments (Fig. 28). The destructive wavelengths correspond to the zones of absorption for the purines and pyrimidines. Grafts between an anucleate and a nucleate fragment showed that the morphogenetic substances stored in the anucleate fragment are destroyed by UV irradiation, since this fragment, when

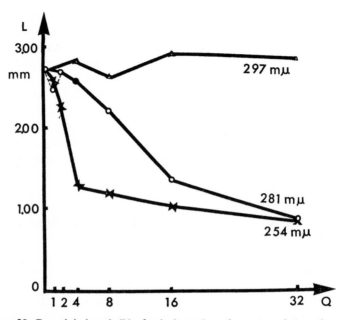

Figure 28. Growth in length (L) of apical anucleate fragments of *A. mediterranea* irradiated with uv, as a function of the dose, Q, of irradiation for variable wavelengths. (After Six, 1956a.)

irradiated, loses all influence on the form of the cap (Werz and Hämmerling, 1961). Taking into account the effective wavelengths and the results concerning the RNAs, these substances would seem to be destroyed in the cytoplasm by irradiation.

Effectively, irradiation with ultraviolet rays inhibits the cytoplasmic incorporation of ^{14}C-adenine and ^{3}H-uridine, especially in the apical zone where this incorporation is usually stronger, whether the algae as a whole or simply the rhizoid is irradiated. On the other hand, when only the apex is irradiated, labelling of the rhizoids with the above precursors is actually increased. This is also true for ^{35}S-methionine and for the sulphur proteins, which, as we have seen, behave in the same way as the cytoplasmic RNAs of nuclear origin (Brachet and Olszewska, 1960; Olszewska et al., 1961).

Penetrating ultraviolet radiation therefore seems generally to attack the cytoplasm, destroying at least part of the RNAs there, and particularly those which come from the nucleus; the latter is subsequently able to furnish a new supply of morphogenetic substances so that the irradiated algae regenerate nevertheless in a normal way. High labelling of the rhizoids when the apical zone alone is irradiated must therefore imply nuclear 'emissions' which tend to compensate for cytoplasmic losses.

These findings contrast with the results of X-ray irradiation, which always affect the cytoplasm, but also attack the nucleus itself, with consequent repercussions on morphogenetic capacity.

(c) GAMMA RADIATIONS

High doses of gamma radiations inhibit cap formation in *Acetabularia*; cellular regeneration and cyst formation are even more radiosensitive. These observations suggest that processes which require new synthesis of morphogenetic substances are most affected by radiation. Autoradiographic studies confirm this hypothesis: ^{3}H-uracil incorporation is strongly inhibited by radiation while ^{3}H-leucine incorporation remains unaffected or is only slightly decreased. Bonotto et al. (1970) have concluded that gamma rays affect transcription, i.e. RNA synthesis, more than translation i.e., protein synthesis.

2. Chemical inhibitors

According to the biochemical analyses, protein synthesis in the anucleate fragments was not immediately inhibited by enucleation, whereas, on the contrary, RNA synthesis was much more affected, though not entirely eliminated. For this reason, it seemed interesting to carry out further studies at this level.

(a) THE ACTION OF RIBONUCLEASE

Nucleate and anucleate algae were placed in sea water containing ribonuclease (1 mg/ml); the enzyme probably enters the algae since growth and morphogenesis are stopped in two types of algal stalk (Fig. 29). This arrest is irreversible for anucleate fragments; the nucleate halves, on the other hand, are able to recommence normal development without any apparent anomaly as soon as they are replaced in normal

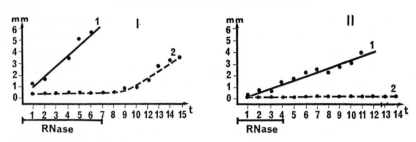

Figure 29. Growth in length of the nucleate (I) and the anucleate (II) fragments of *Acetabularia* placed in normal medium (1) or in a medium containing ribonuclease (2). At the beginning of the experiment, the nucleate fragments measured 3 mm and the anucleate fragments 10 mm. *Abcissa*: time in days. *Ordinate*: elongation in mm. (After Stich and Plant, 1958.)

culture medium (Stich and Plaut, 1958; de Vitry, 1962b). Puiseux-Dao (1958a, 1962) obtained identical results with the same and a neighbouring species, *Batophora oerstedii*.

Protein synthesis is inhibited, if only to a limited extent, by this treatment, as is proved by the estimations made by Stich and Plaut (1958): the total protein content of the algae remains constant (instead of increasing) in the presence of ribonuclease given for four to seven days, and increases after the experiment, at least in nucleate algae. The assay technique used failed to detect any protein synthesis in the fragments without a nucleus, under these conditions. But in fact, ^{14}C-phenylalanine or ^{14}C-lysine can be incorporated by both types of *Acetabularia* fragments after sojourn in a medium containing the enzyme studied (Brachet and Six, 1966). A stimulation of protein synthesis may be observed and seems to be associated with a rise in RNA content, which is higher in the treated than in the control algae, whether they are nucleate or anucleate. There is probably a correlation between this increase in RNA and the fact that in *Batophora*, treatment with ribonuclease provokes a definite nuclear reaction, with intense stimulation of nuclear 'emissions' (Puiseux-Dao, 1958a). Protein synthesis is activated not only in the hyaloplasm, but also in the chloroplasts (Brachet and Six, 1966). Effectively, these pathways in plastid synthesis must be affected, since a similar effect has also been reported for another alga, a *Mougeotia* species: the chloroplast lamellae tend to disappear at the beginning of the treatments, while at a later stage their formation is, conversely, strongly stimulated, especially if the material is replaced in a normal culture medium (Puiseux-Dao, 1964).

Taken as a whole, these results permit the supposition that the morphogenesis of whole algae and of their organelles depends on protein syntheses which, themselves, require the presence of RNAs of nuclear and cytoplasmic origin, one or several of which are inactivated by ribonuclease. This inactivation, though not quantitatively high, is generally followed by recuperation involving the stimulation of RNA synthesis and, consequently, of protein synthesis.

(b) THE EFFECTS OF ACTINOMYCIN D

Taking into account the great diversity of the algal RNAs, it became essential to characterise the RNAs of nuclear and cytoplasmic origin which are required for the specific development of the cells. Actinomycins C and D, which block the synthesis of RNAs at transcription level on DNA, therefore became valuable tools for studying this problem.

The addition of actinomycin D, at a concentration of 10 to 20 μg/ml, to the culture medium for periods varying from two days to three weeks, blocks the growth and morphogenesis of whole plants, especially when they are still tiny (10 mm in length). *Acetabularia* which are ready to initiate a cap are much less affected. When treated cells are replaced in a normal medium, their development usually recommences, although this is not always the case; sometimes an ephemeral stimulatory effect is observed (Brachet et al., 1964; Zetsche, 1964a). Morphogenetic substances may include messenger RNAs. If this is so, older plants would inevitably contain a larger store of them than young germlings, and this in itself would explain the lack of effect of the antibiotic at later stages.

When newly amputated nuclear fragments are so treated, being consequently deprived of their apical morphogenetic reserves, striking inhibition of their regeneration is recorded (Brachet et al., 1964; Zetsche, 1964a). Identical results were obtained with actinomycin C by Schweiger and Schweiger (1963). This evidence confirms the involvement of RNAs, which are probably messengers, among the apical morphogenetic substances which originate in the nucleus.

Both actinomycins C and D have but little effect upon anucleate stalks which are already big enough to produce caps (Schweiger and Schweiger, 1963; Zetsche, 1964): the algae grow and caps come to completion, but are nevertheless of smaller dimensions than untreated anucleate controls (Brachet et al., 1964). Here again, experimental findings encourage the assumption that the RNAs controlling morphogenesis are of nuclear origin, and are stored by the apex in sufficiently large quantities to permit cap initiation. Conversely, the growth of the latter probably depends on messengers of cytoplasmic origin, since growth is slowed down or arrested during antibiotic treatment. Moreover, actinomycin D may well inhibit the first stages of the formation of cysts in the reproductive organs (Werz, 1968).

A few diverse experimental findings bring additional evidence in support of this interpretation. For instance, *Acetabularia* which have been maintained in media containing actinomycin for three to four weeks, then cut in two and immediately transferred to normal medium are virtually unable to produce caps. It is therefore feasible to believe that the antibiotic has prevented the elaboration of an apical stock of messenger RNAs (Brachet et al., 1964). Similarly, uninucleate grafts previously treated with actinomycin between the species *mediterranea* and *crenulata* (*medi-creno*) tend towards the dominant expression of morphological features characteristic of *crenulata*, whereas untreated control grafts display only traces of the characteristics of this species (Zetsche, 1964).

Cytological observations reveal considerable alteration of the nucleus and of the plastids in the presence of the antibiotic (page 44); these cell organelles are indeed the two main sites of template DNA activity in *Acetabularia* so that this finding constitutes further experimental evidence in favour of an arrest of the synthesis of messenger RNAs. Nucleolar function seems to be especially susceptible, as in all the materials studied, and in the algae, as elsewhere, inhibition probably primordially concerns the formation of ribosomal RNAs (Attardi et al., 1967; Scherrer et al., 1967).

Autoradiographic evidence is equally convincing and convergent. Effectively, actinomycin enters the cell and binds rapidly to cytoplasmic sites. It accumulates in the perinuclear zone, becoming detectable in the nucleus only after a latent period of about forty-eight hours, although serious malformations of the latter organelles are already visible after twenty-four hours of treatment. Furthermore, the antibiotic alters the level of incorporation of the labelled nucleosides: ^{3}H-uridine and ^{3}H-guanosine into *Acetabularia* (de Vitry, 1965c). Enzymatic tests were used in each case to control the nature of the molecules into which the precursors had been incorporated, and the general plan of the experiments followed one of the two general plans which follow.

(i) The algae were labelled in the dark in the presence of actinomycin D, in order to study its effects on the synthesis of messenger RNAs *in situ* (treatments varied in duration from four to ten days).

(ii) Incorporations were permitted for a period of two and a half hours, during which time the nucleus became labelled; the algae were then transferred to non-radioactive medium containing actinomycin, in the light, to see whether the antibiotic would influence the transfer of nuclear RNAs towards the apex.

Respectively, the results obtained were as follows.

(i) Incorporation of nucleosides into the nucleolus is completely inhibited by actinomycin, while the nucleoplasm is much less affected. Radioactivity is diminished sharply in the perinuclear zone, while, in a general way, the labelling of the cytoplasm is relatively less sensitive (Fig. 30). Identical results were obtained with whole algae and with nucleate fragments. The evidence demonstrates the preferential sensitivity of the nucleolus to actinomycin, in good agreement with the biochemical results indicating that this antibiotic initially acts upon ribosomal biogenesis (Attardi et al., 1967; Scherrer et al., (1967). However, the synthesis of other RNAs, doubtless messenger RNAs, is also prevented by actinomycin; and this phenomenon may also be responsible for the overall decrease in the labelling of the treated algae. The formation of RNAs in the cytoplasm is probably less affected than the syntheses which occur in the nucleus.

(ii) Whereas nuclear radioactivity in the control algae diminishes only very slowly, that of the cytoplasm and, particularly, that of the apex, increases; algae placed in a medium to which actinomycin has been added lose label from the nucleus, and radioactivity accumulates at the base of the axial stalks. Thus, the movement of RNAs from the nucleus into the cytoplasm is still possible, but instead of migrating towards the morphogenetic zone, these molecules tend to accumulate in the basal part of the cell (Fig. 30).

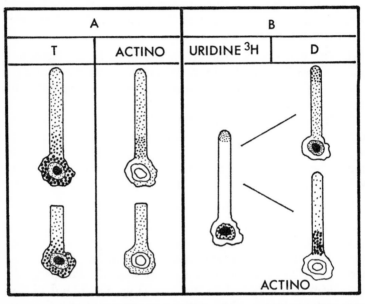

Figure 30. Study of the incorporation of ³H-uridine and of its mobility in *A. mediterranea* in the dark (A) and in the light (B). (A) Labelling of the nucleate fragments and of whole algae: Left, in the control; right, in the presence of actinomycin. (B) Left, ordinary short labelling; top right, chase (D) in the control; bottom right, in the presence of actinomycin. (After de Vitry, 1965.)

Actinomycin, as has been seen, had little quick effect on the incorporation of radioactive amino acids. However, when the algae have undergone pretreatment with the antibiotic, before labelling, a drop in nuclear radioactivity is recorded, when the precursors used are tryptophan and, especially, arginine (de Vitry, 1965c). This reduced incorporation is probably due to the cessation of the synthesis of ribosomes.

Altogether, this data concerning actinomycin and its effects on *Acetabularia*, lead to the conclusion that this substance inhibits morphogenesis by a triple mechanism.

(i) The main effect involves a reduction in ribosome formation characterised by changes in nucleolar morphology and by a loss of synthetic activity by that organelle, made manifest by reduced labelling with nucleosides. This major effect has relatively slow repercussion on the apical morphogenesis of the alga.

(ii) The synthesis is reduced in the nucleoplasm of messenger RNAs which could be responsible for morphogenesis proper; their transfer from the base to the apex of the stalk is also inhibited.

(iii) A very slight fall in the synthesis of cytoplasmic RNAs produced by actinomycin is nevertheless enough to be responsible, particularly in anucleate fragments, for the cessation of growth in *Acetabularia*.

(c) THE ACTION OF PHENYLETHYLALCOHOL (PEA), FLUORODEOXY-URIDINE (FUDR), HYDROXYUREA AND ETHIDIUM BROMIDE

An attempt was made to interfere directly with the synthesis of DNAs and of messenger RNAs. PEA inhibits the synthesis of DNA reversibly in bacteria, and has for this reason been used with *Acetabularia*. FUDR prevents the formation of thymidylic acid by acting specifically on thymidylate synthetase, which catalyses the methylation of deoxyuridylic acid; for this reason, its effects on *Acetabularia* have been analysed. Hydroxyurea is also a very potent inhibitor of the synthesis of DNAs, acting upon the reduction of ribonucleotides to give deoxyribonucleotides.

(i) *The action of phenylethylalcohol* (*de Vitry, 1965b*). Growth of nucleate and anucleate fragments is reversibly arrested by a concentration of 1% of PEA. Both cap and rhizoids present morphological anomalies. However, after a short three-day treatment with PEA, followed by transfer to normal medium stalks lacking nuclei, comprising only the upper two-thirds of the alga, show not only stimulated growth but also the formation of caps and even of rhizoids. It should be noted that the formation of rhizoids is quite exceptional in control anucleate cultures and the effect of PEA can therefore only be due to the potentialisation of some factor which is repressed in untreated, normal anucleate fragments.

Nuclear volume is considerably reduced by PEA; auto-radiography shows parallel reduction in the incorporation of ³H-thymidine into the nucleus and cytoplasm of the algae. ³H-uridine incorporation is similarly restrained in every sector of the cell. As regards ¹⁴C-lysine incorporation, differential results are obtained: inhibition is observed to be complete in the nucleus, whereas the cytoplasm is but little affected or, in the apical zone, shows slight increase.

Taken together, all these results obtained with a single dose of PEA, seem to bring conclusive evidence of the inhibition of the synthesis of DNA. Consequently, RNA anabolism is also stopped, it seems. As a further result, anomalies of growth and morphogenesis occur, doubtless associated with disturbed protein synthesis.

(ii) *The action of 5-fluorodeoxyuridine (de Vitry, 1965b).* Complete inhibition of the morphogenesis of nucleate *Acetabularia* is produced by high concentrations (10^{-3}M), partial inhibition by low concentrations (10^{-4}M). More striking effects are observed in freshly excised nucleate fragments than in whole algae. Although anucleate fragments are less affected, they nevertheless bear caps which develop various anomalies. The addition of thymidine, uridine or, most particularly, orotic acid, exert a protective effect upon algae submitted to this anti-metabolite. Nuclear aspect is changed by treatment with FUDR, one of the most striking effects being the increase in basophilia.

Lower levels of ³H-thymidine incorporation than in controls are recorded after (not during) treatment of nucleate fragments with FUDR (10^{-3}M) for three days, except in the nucleoplasm, where an accumulation of the radioisotope is recorded. On the contrary, as compared with anucleate untreated controls, anucleate fragments exhibit lower levels of labelling in every part of the cell.

These findings permit the author to suggest that, as is the case in bacteria, FUDR inhibits thymidylate synthetase and does not prevent the use of exogenous thymidine, detectable particularly in the nucleus.

The complicating factor of 'migration' of nuclear RNAs from the basal to the apical end of the alga (page 42) can be avoided if the algae are placed in the dark during study of the metabolism of RNAs in the presence of FUDR. Radioactivity due to ^{3}H-uridine accumulates in the nucleolus both in whole algae and, even more intensely, in nucleate, excised fragments. Clearly, in the presence of this inhibitor, RNA *synthesis* can take place in the nucleus, though the molecules formed may be abnormal, whereas *transfer* of the synthesised RNAs from the nucleus to the perinuclear cytoplasm, is impossible (Fig. 31).

On the basis of these results, it was therefore postulated that if, after the usual three hours' 'pulse' specimens were illuminated during a 'chase' period in the presence of FUDR, it would be possible to analyse the effects of this substance on the *migration* of radioactive nuclear RNAs towards the apical morphogenetically active region. Such experiments result in the maintenance of a fairly high level of nuclear labelling and in an accumulation of radioisotopes at the basal end of the stalk. Thus, FUDR clearly inhibits the transfer of RNAs of nuclear origin towards the apex of *Acetabularia* (Fig. 31).

In anucleate fragments, the presence of FUDR in the culture medium has little effect upon the incorporation of some aminoacids, like lysine, and partially inhibits the incorporation of others, like tryptophan and phenylalanine. In nucleate fragments, on the other hand, this substance actually increases the level of labelling with amino acids, both in the nucleus and the cytoplasm; the stimulatory effect is particularly striking with lysine.

Morphogenetic anomalies and perturbed labelling in algae treated with FUDR permit the thought that this substance does not prevent the incorporation of exogenous thymidine. But, particularly in the nucleus, RNA synthesis is deeply modified and their exodus from that organelle is prevented, perhaps because the molecules formed are abnormal, being synthesised on altered segments of the DNA template. The activation of protein synthesis itself seems difficult to interpret.

(iii) *The action of hydroxyurea* (*Brachet, 1968*). Hydroxyurea, like the above described inhibitors, brings about the cessation

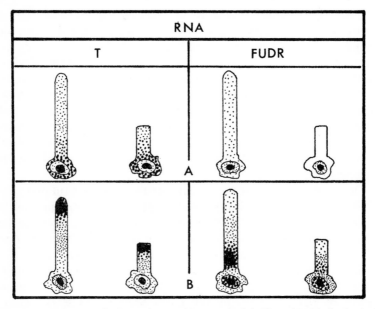

Figure 31. Influence of 5-fluorodeoxyuridine on the labelling of RNAs in the dark
(A) and in the light (B). (T) controls: whole algae and nucleate fragments.
(FUDR) labelling of whole algae in the presence of FUDR (10^{-3} M) or labelling
of nucleate parts of algae after a treatment with FUDR (10^{-4} M; 2 months).
(After de Vitry, 1965.)

of growth and morphogenesis in nucleate and anucleate
fragments treated with concentrations of 100 μg of this substance per ml. Even after one week, this inhibition is still
reversible (Brachet, 1967); it can also be attenuated by the
addition of thymidine or of NADPH. The incorporation of
uridine and thymidine into the nucleic acids of the algae is
decreased, as compared with controls, but the buoyant density
after ultracentrifugation in caesium chloride of DNAs extracted
from the treated material, remains the same (Heilporn and
Limbosch, 1970). The synthesis of DNA is thus, probably,
required for cap formation in *Acetabularia*, even in the anucleate
fragments (Brachet, 1968).

(iv) *The action of ethidium bromide*. Ethidium bromide (EB)
strongly inhibits mitochondrial DNA synthesis and has muta-
genic effects. In the presence of this substance (20–100 μg/ml)
nucleate and anucleate *Acetabularia* lose their hair whorls; both

growth and morphogenesis are stopped. These effects are reversible when algae are returned to sea water but treated plants often form anomalous caps depending on the dose (Heilporn and Limbosch, 1969; Puiseux-Dao and Dazy, 1970). The synthesis of cytoplasmic DNA is reversibly arrested by EB. Even after five days' treatment the mitochondrial peak obtained in CsCl gradients (d = 1,714) disappears almost completely; however, chloroplast DNA (d = 1,704) is always found (Heilporn and Limbosh, 1970). On the electron micrographs of treated *Acetabularia*, three main effects were observed in chloroplasts: the arrangement of the lamellae is disturbed with high doses, the DNA fibrils and the ribosomes are condensed and the plastidal stroma appears to be more or less empty; many figures interpreted as division stages are present; the mitochondria seem less numerous (Dazy, in preparation).

(d) THE ACTION OF PUROMYCIN AND CYCLOHEXIMIDE

(i) *The action of puromycin.* Puromycin, an analog of transfer RNAs, inhibits protein synthesis at ribosome level. When used at low concentrations (10 μg/ml) it has little effect upon *Acetabularia*; both nucleate and anucleate fragments acquire a yellow hue, however, especially towards the apex. Reproductive caps are extremely abnormal in their presence (Plate 12). Higher concentrations of puromycin added to the culture medium (15 to 20 μg/ml) stop growth and morphogenesis altogether. In the case of anucleate parts, inhibition may become irreversible, after a variable number of days treatment. Algae containing a nucleus are able, on the other hand, to recommence development under such conditions after a variable period of latency. Numerous heteromorphoses are observed, then, especially if treatment has been effectuated under dark conditions, the algae develop bifid or trifid stalks (Brachet et al., 1964). These observations led Brachet to the conclusion that the ordered synthesis of proteins is disturbed by puromycin.

Since this substance totally prevents growth and development, it is feasible to imagine that it causes the accumulation of morphogenetic substances in the cytoplasm of treated cells. Indeed, when *Acetabularia* sojourns in a medium containing 30 μg of puromycin/ml for a period of about ten days before being transferred to normal medium after excision of the basal part containing the nucleus, the anucleate fragments are equivalent to anucleate untreated *Acetabularia*. Therefore as far as morphogenetic capacity is concerned, their development is simply a few days behind that of controls. The nucleus must therefore have supplied morphogenetic substances during the treatment (Zetsche, 1965). Correlation of these findings with the effects of darkness on *Acetabularia* bring this author to the conclusion that morphogenetic substances accumulate in the perinuclear region (page 41). The behaviour of anucleate parts maintained for ten days in darkness, or of algae treated with puromycin for an equivalent period, is exactly the same if they are enucleated at the time of transfer to normal culture medium (Fig. 32). To all intents and purposes, the estimation of total protein content in both types of experiment (Zetsche, 1966a) establishes the static, arrested nature of protein synthesis during the period of puromycin treatment, and the immediate increase in protein content when the algae are replaced in normal solution. Zetsche (1965) has, moreover, treated uni-nucleate fragments hybridising *crenulata* and *mediterranea* (*crenₒ-medᵢ*) with puromycin at a concentration of 50 μg/ml for twenty-four hours, just after the achievement of the graft: cap formation was found to be retarded. Removal of the *mediter-*

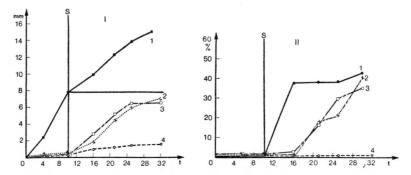

Figure 32. (I) Elongation of anucleate fragments derived from *A. mediterranea* treated with puromycin or placed in the dark before sectioning (S). (1) Controls (non-amputated). (2) Anucleate fragments coming from algae treated with 30 μg of puromycin per ml. (3) Anucleate fragments coming from algae kept in the dark. (4) Anucleate fragments replaced in the presence of puromycin after enucleation. *Abcissa*: time in days. *Ordinate*: elongation in mm. (II) Percentage of caps formed by the anucleate fragments placed in the same conditions as the preceding ones. (After Zetsche, 1965a.)

ranea nucleus from these grafts, after ten days treatment, results in caps expressing mostly *mediterranea* character, whereas control grafts, enucleated at the same time but not treated with puromycin, form caps resembling *crenulata* more closely in their morphology, as is normally the case. Proof is thus obtained that during the period of puromycin treatment, the nucleus of the *mediterranea* species has continued to synthesise morphogenetic substances which have migrated into the cytoplasm of the *creno-medi* cells.

Finally, if 10 μg actinomycin/ml are added at the same time as puromycin to the experimental solution, the morphogenetic capacities of the portions lacking a nucleus become very weak, after treatment; these results constitute supplementary evidence in favour of the conclusion that messenger and ribosomal RNAs formed in the nucleus are among the substances responsible for cytoplasmic morphogenesis.

The effects of puromycin have been analysed by autoradiography; labelling was achieved in light and darkness after treatments of variable duration with the antibiotic. Generally, puromycin at a concentration of 30 μg/ml reduces the incorporation of labelled amino-acids: the inhibition may reach 80% as compared with controls, when treatment with the antibiotic has lasted about twelve days (Fig. 33). More than this, ^{3}H-guanosine incorporation into the nucleus of treated algae is strongly enhanced as compared with controls, while the converse is true of the cytoplasm, where labelling is relatively less intense.

All these results can be interpreted in the following way: puromycin inhibits the synthesis of all proteins to a greater or lesser extent. Concomitantly, the amount of RNA in the nucleus increases, reflecting in all probability an accumulation of messenger RNAs and of ribosomal precursors, since the ribosomes remain incomplete in the absence of the required proteins (de Vitry, 1965). The data and the hypotheses advanced to explain them, are in perfect agreement with the findings of Zetsche (1965a, 1966a).

(ii) *The action of cycloheximide.* Cycloheximide (actidione), which acts at the level of the transfer RNAs, inhibits the synthesis of proteins in a way which is fairly analogous to the effects of puromycin, and its action on morphogenesis is also

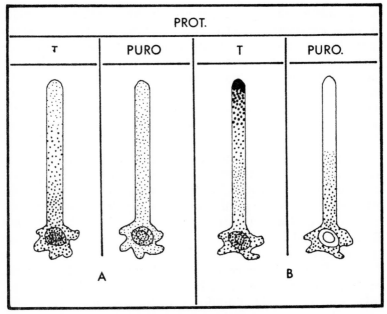

Figure 33. Influence of puromycin on the incorporation of ^{14}C-lysine in whole *A. mediterranea* in the dark (A) or in the light (B). (T) controls; (Puro) algae treated with puromycin before labelling. (After de Vitry, 1965.)

very similar to that observed with the latter substance (Brachet, 1967c).

As one would expect, all inhibition of protein synthesis affects both nucleate and anucleate fragments, without preventing the synthesis of messenger and ribosomal RNAs of nuclear origin required for morphogenesis, at least for a certain time, so that these substances accumulate in the cytoplasm and can be used when treatment with the inhibitor has ceased. The anomalies observed in algae without nuclei replaced in normal medium after treatments with puromycin, suggest that some synthetic pathways are more sensitive than others, and an attempt has therefore been made to inhibit some of them in a preferential way, using amino acid analogs.

(e) THE ACTION OF DIFFERENT ANTIMETABOLITES OF AMINO ACIDS

In view of the attention given to nucleocytoplasmic interrelations in *Acetabularia* and also because the results obtained

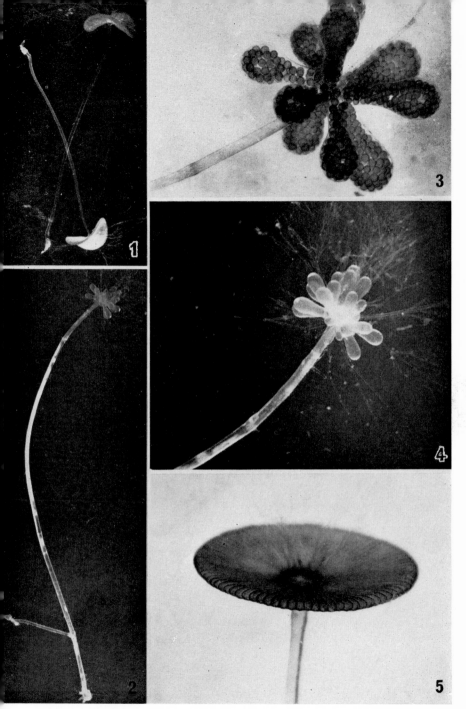

Plate 11. Grafts between *A. mediterranea* and *A. peniculus.* (1) *A. mediter-*
ranea ($\times 1.5$). (2) Graft with intermediate cap ($\times 2$). (3), (4) and (5)
Details of the caps: (3) *A. peniculus* cap. (4) Intermediate cap. (5) *A.*
mediterranea cap ($\times 5$). (Puiseux-Dao, unpublished.)

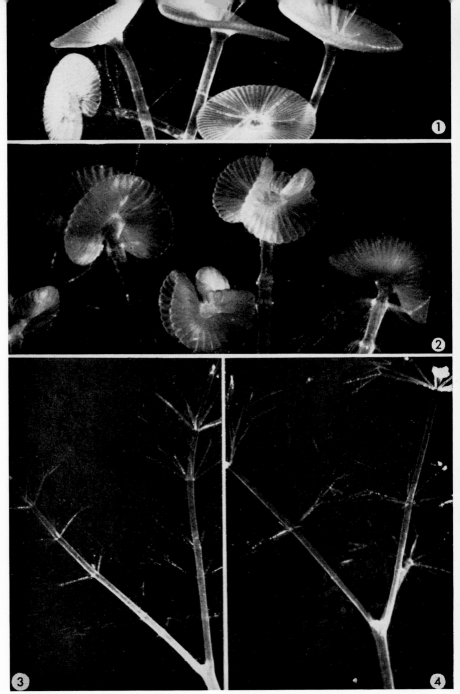

Plate 12. (1) Reproductive caps of *A. mediterranea* (controls). (2) Reproductive caps of *A. mediterranea* treated with low concentrations (5 μg/ml) of puromycin. (3) and (4) Bifid and trifid algae obtained in the presence of strong concentrations (30 μm/gl) of puromycin for two weeks ($\times 3$). (After Brachet et al., 1964; photos, Brachet.)

by autoradiography using ^{35}S labelled precursors (page 81) and indicating that proteins emanating from the nucleus accumulate in the apical zone during morphogenesis, the first antimetabolite for amino acid incorporation was *ethionine*.

Ethionine (10^{-3}M) seems to stimulate the formation of caps in anucleate fragments, but many of these reproductive organs are morphologically abnormal; on the other hand, regeneration of nuclear fragments is strongly inhibited (Brachet, 1958a,b, de Vitry, 1962b). Since autoradiography using ^{35}S-methionine has demonstrated the important part played by sulphur proteins in morphogenesis, other inhibitors of sulphur metabolism have also been studied.

Beta-mercaptoethanol (M/300) prevents the appearance of caps in both types of fragments (nucleate and anucleate): the algae take on the appearance of plants grown in subnormal light conditions (Beth, 1953a) or in starvation conditions (such as, for instance, in pure sea water: Dao, 1954a). M/100 *dithiodiglycol* stimulates the morphogenesis of reproductive caps in the anucleate parts, whereas mercaptoethanol-ethylgluconamide inhibits their formation, though less completely than mercaptoethanol itself, and induces malformations at the same time. No reproductive organs are formed at all in the presence of lipoic acid (Brachet, 1962). Selenium in the form of SeO_4^{2-} instead of SO_4^{2-} inhibits growth and morphogenesis reversibly in nucleate, irreversibly in anucleate fragments. Uninucleate grafts between anucleate *crenulata* treated with selenium and untreated *mediterranea* furnishes caps resembling *mediterranea* much more than controls. Thus, selenium acts as an antimetabolite in perturbing the metabolism of sulphur proteins, the morphogenetic role of which is once more demonstrated (Werz, 1961b). Brachet has drawn the conclusion that the — SH $\rightleftharpoons$ — SS — balance is very important for morphogenesis, at the membrane level, and Clauss (1961) has effectively shown that ^{35}S is very intensely incorporated by developing membranes. However, this question has not been adequately studied, not even the incorporation of sulphur compounds by the algae has been investigated (Werz, 1963c).

When *p-fluorophenylalanine* is added to sea-water (10 to 50 μg/ml), it immediately inhibits the development of both nucleate and anucleate *Acetabularia*, but this analog has

8—AACB * *

relatively little effect upon the formation of sterile whorls, whereas it completely stops the morphogenesis of caps. Phenylalanine and tyrosine protect the algae against this selective inhibitory effect. Further, the action of the analog is reversible so long as the algae are replaced in normal medium before the normally cultured controls have initiated caps; conversely, if the transfer is only effectuated when the controls have already formed their caps, the treated *Acetabularia* remain incapable of forming reproductive organs even after their return to a solution deprived of the inhibitor (Zetsche, 1966b).

These data permit the conclusion that the sulphur proteins play an important role in the morphogenesis of *Acetabularia* and, further, that the completion of the reproductive caps requires at least some proteins which differ from those necessary for axial extension.

Convergent results are thus obtained from all the experiments involving inhibitors of the pathway DNA—RNAs—proteins, and inspire the following conclusions.

The nucleus is an active centre for the synthesis of both messenger and ribosomal RNAs which are responsible, at least in part, for the morphogenesis of *Acetabularia*. These substances, associated with proteins, move into the cytoplasm where they can be stored for a certain length of time. They control the syntheses required first of all for axial extension of the stalk carrying sterile whorls, and then for the genesis of a reproductive cap. Essential for both these morphogenetic processes is the synthesis not only of proteins under nuclear control but also, most probably, of others under the control of satellite extranuclear DNAs. The elaboration and the regulation of the biochemical pathways leading successively to each type of morphological achievement in one single cell represents a complex group of problems which can be approached in several ways.

D. REGULATION OF PROTEIN SYNTHESIS

The morphogenetic, biochemical and autoradiographical findings in *Acetabularia* suggest that the pool of messengers of nuclear origin have an average life duration of about two to three weeks. Because of this, attempts were made to discover whether messengers leaving the nucleus together are translated simultaneously in the cytoplasm, or sequentially, and whether there is any temporal variation in the type of message transmitted. The possible normal control of the regulation of metabolism was also studied. These two approaches used in the study of the regulation of protein synthesis are outlined below.

1. Sequential translation of nuclear messages as a function of time

The morphogenesis of *Acetabularia* involves two consecutive phases: the formation and extension of the cylindrical axis, followed by the genesis of a reproductive cap. The morphogenetic substances are stocked in the tip of the algae (page 54) and it is therefore possible to excise the upper segment of the cells to obtain nuclear fragments lacking their preformed stock of nuclear messages. Using nucleate fragments restricted to the basal rhizoid region, Zetsche (1966d) attempted to see whether the messengers required for cap morphogenesis were sent into the cytoplasm as soon as the stalk began to regenerate. To this end, batches of fragments were treated with actinomycin at a concentration of 10 μg/ml either immediately after excision of the stalks or one, two, three and up to fifteen days after this operation. In every case, the sojourn in actinomycin was stopped forty-seven days after the beginning of the experiment: the number of caps which had been formed was then counted. In the regenerating fragments, apical messenger RNAs originating in the nucleus can only have been synthesised after excision, while the last to be synthesised must have been formed before actinomycin treatment began. Since the untreated controls take about fifteen days to regenerate a stalk before the cap initiates, it might be thought that during this initial period only messages concerning stalk formation would be issued by the nucleus. In reality, this is probably not the case, since nucleate parts placed in medium containing actinomycin from the third day after excision of the stalk onwards, formed cap rudiments in 35% of cases; when the antibiotic is added on the sixth day after amputation of the stalk, 66% of the algae produce a more or less well developed reproductive organ (Fig. 34).

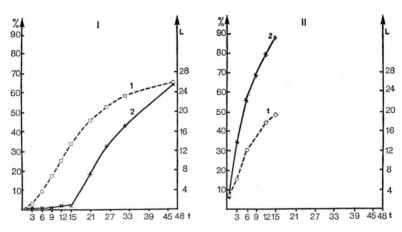

Figure 34. Study of the regeneration of nucleate fragments of *A. mediterranea* 0, 3, 6, 9, 12 or 15 days after removal of apical part of the algae. 47 days later, the extension (elongation) of the fragment was measured (L) and the percentage of caps formed was estimated (%). (I) Evolution of the control fragments during an experiment lasting 47 days. (1) Elongation of fragments; (2) Percentage of caps formed during the same experimental period. (II) At the end of 47 days of regeneration, aspect of the fragments placed in the presence of actinomycin (10 μg/ml): 0, 3, 6, 9, 12 or 15 days after amputation of the apical part of the algae. *Abcissa*: time in days after beginning of treatment. *Ordinate*: percentage of caps formed after 47 days (2); *ordinate L*: elongation after 47 days (1).

Clearly, the messenger RNAs which control cap initiation and morphogenesis are formed in the nucleus at the same time as those required for stalk regeneration. They are probably stocked in the apical zone without being immediately 'translated', unless the proteins formed on translation are themselves conserved in an inactive form. Further, the more the treatment with actinomycin is retarded, the greater is the diameter of the cap. This finding is not at variance with the opinion expressed by Brachet (1964), who thinks that while cap *initiation* is certainly controlled by the nucleus, cap *growth* depends on the functioning, rather of the cytoplasmic DNAs.

When the delay before the appearance of a cap is studied in *Acetabularia* about to reach maturity, divided into three batches: controls, algae treated with actinomycin and algae from which the rhizoid containing the nucleus has been excised; the controls are seen to form caps later than the other two batches of algae. This could be interpreted as meaning that the translation of RNAs responsible for cap initiation is normally inhibited by substances of nuclear origin which exert a repressor effect (Beth, 1953b; Zetsche, 1966d).

2. Cytoplasmic regulation of the activity of cytoplasmic enzymes

Obviously, the simplest hypothesis would consist in suggesting that the nucleus controls the different stages of morphogenesis by controlling the pool of enzymes in the cell. This is why research into the regulation of enzyme action and synthesis has been started in *Acetabularia*, beginning with the study of the phosphatases (Spencer and Harris, 1964). After having demonstrated that *Acetabularia crenulata* contains at least three phosphatases having different pH optima (5, 8·5 and 12), all of which are synthesised even in the absence of the nucleus, they also found that the enzyme active at pH 12 only appears a very short while before cap initiation, not only in whole algae but also in nucleate and anucleate fragments. The implication of these findings is that enzyme synthesis does not occur simultaneously, even if the coordinating messages are emitted by the nucleus at the same time: the regulation of translation therefore probably occurs in the cytoplasm.

Zetsche (1966c) reached the same conclusion after studying the synthesis of UDP-glucose$_4$-epimerase. Indeed, the membrane of *Acetabularia* contains mainly mannose, glucose and rhamnose, but the axial stalk, particularly rich in mannose and almost lacking in rhamnose, differs in sugar content from the membrane of the cap, which contains more glucose, galactose and rhamnose (Werz, 1963c; Zetsche, 1967). First of all this author showed the existence of enzymes required for the synthesis of the above mentioned hexoses, using fructose, which is abundant in these algae, as a substrate (Zetsche, 1965b, 1966b). Then he followed the evolution of the activity of UDP-glucose$_4$-epimerase in nucleate and anucleate fragments. Effectively, in both of them, just before and during the elaboration of the reproductive organs, a striking increase in the activity of this enzyme is recorded. Since puromycin and actidione (cycloheximide) totally prevent the rise in content of this enzyme, one is really considering protein synthesis, which recommences when antibiotic treatment is brought to an end. Here again, these results imply the sequential translation of messages sent out simultaneously from the nucleus. UDPG-pyrophosphorylase (Fig. 35) behaves exactly like UDP-glucose$_4$-epimerase (Zetsche, 1968, 1969a). The activity of this enzyme increases as morphogenesis of the cap progresses, both in

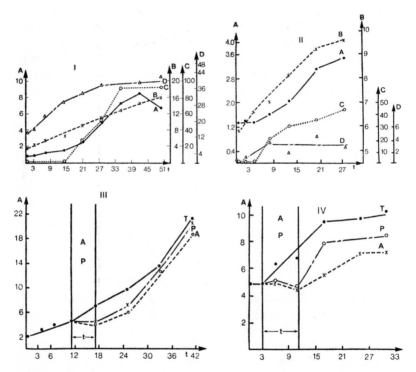

Figure 35. (I) Evolution of the UDPG—pyrophosphorylase activity of nucleate fragments of *A. mediterranea* (A) Enzyme activity in milliunities per plant. (B) quantity of protein nitrogen in μg per plant; (C) percentage of caps formed; (D) average increase in length of the algae, (t) time in days. (II) Evolution of the UDPG-pyrophosphorylase activity of anucleate fragments of *A. mediterranea*. (III) Evolution of the UDPG-pyrophosphorylase activity of nucleate fragments of *A. mediterranea*, in the presence of actidione or of puromycin and after treatment with one of these antibiotics. The treatment (t) has been carried out between the 11th and the 17th day. (T) control; (P) puromycin; (A) actidione. (IV) Evolution of the UDPG-pyrophosphorylase activity of anucleate fragments of *A. mediterranea* in the presence of actidione or of puromycin and after treatment with one of these antibiotics. The treatment (t) has been carried on the 3rd and the 11th day. (After Zetsche, 1968.)

anucleate stalks and in nucleate fragments. Puromycin and actidione provoke a reversible fall in the activity of this enzyme, while actinomycin only affects the basal nucleate fragment undergoing regeneration. The regulation of the activity of this enzyme must also be cytoplasmic.

The control of enzyme synthesis has also been studied by trying to vary the chemical composition of the medium. Nucleate and anucleate algae grown in normally enriched sea water have been compared with similar fragments grown in the same medium, but deficient in phosphate. The result of a transfer from normal to deficient medium is always a reduction in total acid phosphatase activity. This decrease is temporary in whole algae and in nucleate fragments, but permanent in anucleate fragments. The phenomenon is not a simple one. It has been found by electrophoretic analysis, which separates out the three principal isoenzymes, that the drop in activity which is observed is only due to one of these isoenzymes, localised in the plastids. What is more, the secondary increase in phosphatase activity which only occurs in the presence of the nucleus, seems to be associated with isoenzyme 1, which is also plastidial. With regard to the nucleus, this isoenzyme, taking into account the fact that there is a latent period lasting several days, acts as a repressible enzyme. It should also be mentioned that this problem is rendered even more complex in *Acetabularia* by the presence in the algae of polyphosphates (page 37) which are hydrolysed in algae placed in medium deficient in phosphate; moreover, the polyphosphates also disappear from both nucleate and anucleate halves when *Acetabularia* is cut in two (Brachet and Lievens, 1968; Brachet, in press). However, it remains plausible to think that the synthesis of certain plastid proteins, including isoenzyme 1, is under nuclear control which is consistent with the pattern given by Puiseux-Dao (1970) for the nuclear control of plastidal functions.

3. The role of hormones in Acetabularia

Comparisons have been made of the effects of *indoleacetic acid* (*IAA*) and of *naphthalene acetic acid* (*NAA*) on the growth and morphogenesis of whole algae and anucleate fragments. These substances, which are inactive at low concentrations, and inhibitory at high concentrations, particularly in the case of NAA, cause an acceleration of extension of the stalk at concentrations varying from 10^{-6} to 10^{-5} (Dao, 1954b), indoleacetic acid being the most active. In the latter case, the reaction of the algae cultivated in sea water is extremely high and one may wonder whether, in this minimal medium, there may not have been an accumulation of RNA and protein precursors, as in algae kept in darkness, and that in the presence of auxin, these would be more rapidly used up.

Thimann and Beth (1955) showed moreover that these auxins are able to accelerate the formation of the reproductive caps, their optimal concentration being higher than for growth (IAA:10^{-4}M; NAA:10^{-5}M). *Acetabularia* responds only slowly to the presence of auxins in the medium, the shortest delay being about ten days, and better in sea water enriched only in nitrates and phosphates than in media containing earth extract. The neutral activators, methylindoleacetate and indolacetonitrile give similar delayed effects, and it is therefore unlikely that pH interferes by slowing down the penetration of these substances (Thimann and Beth, 1959). The amplitude of the reaction which follows the addition of auxins to the culture medium, depends on the metabolic state of the algae and in particular, on the seasonal rhythm when the plants come directly from nature (Dao, 1954b). In impoverished media (pure sea water for instance) IAA is active on growth at concentrations 100 times higher than those which are normally efficient; in such cases, tryptophan is probably used as a source of nitrogen. In every case, the effects described occur in anucleate fragments, suggesting that the intracellular site of action of the auxins is purely cytoplasmic (Thimann and Beth, 1959).

Giberellin also improves the growth of *Acetabularia* at an optimum concentration of 10^{-7} to 10^{-6}M. Like the hormones mentioned above, it also accelerates the morphogenesis of the cap, but at an effective concentration which is higher (10^{-4}M) than the one required to stimulate increase in length. In this case, fertile algae having a short axis are obtained. In the absence of the nucleus, similar effects are produced by giberellin, though on a smaller scale (Zetsche, 1963).

Kinetin also produces such effects, not only in *Acetabularia mediterranea* (Zetsche, 1963), but also in *Acetabularia crenulata*. The concentrations which stimulate growth most efficiently are 10^{-8} to 10^{-7}M, much higher concentrations being inhibitory (10^{-5} and 10^{-4}M). There again, the initiation and formation of the reproductive cap is stimulated by concentrations above those which improve extension (10^{-9} to 10^{-4}M); the caps so produced are small, but of characteristic shape for the species. If the hormone is used on small plants measuring only about 7 mm, the effects of kinetin are all the clearer; long, adult algae having attained 25 mm in length are much less responsive (Spencer, 1968), and the effect of kinetin on them is almost nil. Anucleate fragments react like whole algae, irrespective of having been kept in darkness before enucleation in order to increase their morphogenetic capacity. However, only the apical parts which are capable of morphogenesis are able to give positive results, the basal parts remaining insensitive to the hormone, the site of action of which must therefore be cytoplasmic.

Finally, the appearance of phosphatase activity at pH 12, linked to the biogenesis of the reproductive organs, does not seem to be very sensitive to the action of kinetin.

2-3-5-*triiodobenzoic acid* (Thimann and Beth, 1959) inhibits morphogenesis and the synthesis of alkaline phosphatase (Spencer, 1968) in a reproducible way at the concentrations used (10^{-6} and 10^{-4}M).

Plant hormones seem therefore to have rather irregular and limited effects in *Acetabularia*, and for this reason they may well be absent from normal algae or, perhaps, play only a secondary role. Their site of action, determined experimentally, is in any case cytoplasmic.

E. CONCLUSIONS

The purpose of many investigations has been to analyse the relationship between nucleus and cytoplasm in *Acetabularia*; the situation has been found to be more and more complex as the studies advance. The most conclusive results seem to be the following.

(i) The nucleus is the main site of synthesis of the cell's RNAs; it also synthesises proteins. However, the synthesis of cytoplasmic RNAs seems to play an important role.

(ii) The nucleus sends into the cytoplasm substances which control morphogenesis; these substances, which accumulate in the apical zone of the algae, include RNAs and basic proteins rich in sulphur.

(iii) These RNAs, the synthesis of which is sensitive to actinomycin, include messenger RNAs as well as a high quantity of ribosomal RNAs; at least a part of the sulphur containing basic proteins are probably ribosomal proteins. Together, these substances constitute the cytoplasmic polysomes, most abundant at the apex of the alga.

(iv) In the dark, this pool of nuclear substances leaves the nucleus and migrates first into the perinuclear zone: its further migration into the cytoplasm is slowed down. Stored in this region, the morphogenetic substances are inactive. Puromycin causes a similar accumulation of morphogenetic substances in the algae.

(v) Messages sent simultaneously into the cytoplasm by the nucleus are not all 'translated' at the same time, some being active immediately, others being stored. Regulation of the sequential reading of the nuclear messages takes place in the cytoplasm, with the aid of proteins, some of which may themselves originate in the nucleus.

(vi) The cytoplasm strongly influences the metabolism of the nucleus, but this aspect of nucleocytoplasmic relations is still little known.

(vii) In the cytoplasm, relatively autonomous functional centres exist: these are the mitochondria and the chloroplasts which contain their own DNA and could, at least, intervene in the general phenomena involving cell growth, even if they only do so by way of the synthesis of carbon chains and of the ATP molecules supplying energy for metabolism.

6

The chloroplasts of *Acetabularia* and their functional periodicity

Acetabularia, like all plants, contains at least two kinds of organelles containing satellite DNA: these are the plastids and the mitochondria. The chloroplasts are so numerous that they account for a high proportion of the dry weight of the alga; they are at present the subject of a great deal of research.

A. METABOLIC AUTONOMY OF THE CHLOROPLASTS

1. Nature and replication of the DNA of the chloroplasts

The idea that the plastids of plant cells contain DNA was not at first readily accepted. Since the nucleus and the chloroplasts of the higher plants have very similar buoyant densities, it seemed very possible that chloroplast fractions were simply contaminated by the presence of nuclei or nuclear fragments. Conclusive evidence was supplied when Baltus and Brachet (1962, 1963), as well as Gibor and Izawa (1963), carried out estimations on sedimented plastids isolated from anucleate fragments of *Acetabularia*, using refined fluorimetric techniques. Since then, ultrastructural evidence has also been provided (page 44). More recently, Green et al. (1967, 1970) in Brachet's laboratory, succeeded in characterising the DNA of the chloroplasts and of the mitochondria by CsCl gradient ultra-centrifugation in caesium chloride. Taking into account the possibility of contamination with microorganisms, these DNAs have buoyant densities of 1·704 g/ml and 1·714 g/ml, corresponding to 45% and 55% respectively. When DNA is extracted from pellets of plastids obtained by sucrose gradient purification, it also has a density of 1·703 g/ml; within the limits of experimental error this finding very convincingly confirms the preceding results (Fig. 36).

When the population of plastids in growing stalks of *Acetabularia* is evaluated by counting, it is found to follow an exponential law (Shephard, 1965a). This has been confirmed by calculation for the plastids of the upper halves of algae by Puiseux-Dao (1968). The DNA of these organelles is therefore probably able to replicate. The cytoplasm of these algae effectively incorporates ³H-thymidine, and the radioactivity detected *in situ* by autoradiographic techniques disappears after treatment with deoxyribonuclease (Brachet, 1958a; Shephard, 1965b; de Vitry, 1965). Moreover, no incorporation of this labelled precursor occurs if labelling is effectuated in the presence of inhibitors of DNA synthesis like phenylethylalcohol or 5-fluorodeoxyuridine (de Vitry, 1965). Plastids continue to multiply in enucleate *Acetabularia* for about a week (Shephard, 1965a; Puiseux-Dao, 1970). In the same way, the duplication of DNA seems to be only slightly affected by the removal of the nucleus, especially during the first few days which follow excision, as shown by autoradiography using ³H-thymidine (de Vitry, 1965) and determinations of DNA by fluorimetry (Heilporn-Pohl and Brachet, 1966). Evidence has been obtained by the latter indicating that the amount of DNA in the plastids doubles in five to seven days, measurement which agrees with the temporal results of Shephard (1965a) and with the calculations made by Puiseux-Dao (1968) concerning the duplication of the plastids in the upper sector of the stalk.

Statistically, it has been observed that the farther away from the apices are the plastids, the higher their storage supply; moreover the plastidal thylacoids become very scarce when the reserves increase. Most of the plastids present in the rhizoids seem to be relatively inert. The cyclotic movements, which seem to be very active in the axial stalk of the algae, only produce small oscillatory movements of varying amplitude around a central point of equilibrium, in the distribution of the plastids, except in the case of the smallest among them. As a first approximation, it may therefore be assumed that most of the plastids in the basal old part of *Acetabularia* are in fact storage plastids which do not normally divide, whereas those of the

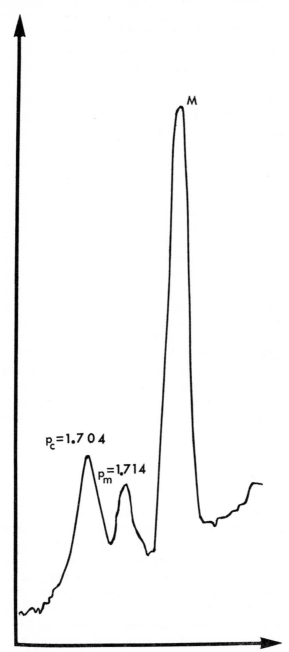

Figure 36. Analysis by gradient centrifugation in CsCl of the DNAs coming from anucleate fragments of *A. mediterranea*. M: DNA of *Micrococcus lysodeikticus* ($\rho = 1\cdot731$ gr/m). (After Green et al., 1967.)

apices contain less polysaccharides but are able to divide. Indeed studies of the plastidal population in the different parts of the algae suggest that there is an apicobasal gradient affecting the division of the chloroplasts. Only in very special circumstances, for instance after excision of the stalk which is followed by the regeneration of the basal fragments, are the basal organelles—or at least some of them—capable of rejuvenating and of dividing; in this way the plastidal population in the new apices rapidly comes to resemble that of a normal apex (Puiseux-Dao and Dazy, 1970). The division of the biggest basal plastids probably occurs by budding. Such budding has been described for basal plastids observed during cap formation by Boloukhère-Presburg (1970). The apicobasal gradient for plastidal division may be under nuclear control; this would explain the slowing down of this process in anucleate fragments (Shephard, 1965a; Puiseux-Dao 1970). The question one is tempted to ask is whether the aging of the plastids, visualised by their polysaccharide content, is related to partial or complete loss of DNA, since Woodcock and Bogorad (1968) have reported considerable variation in the content of DNA in the plastids of *Acetabularia mediterranea*; moreover less DNA areas are visible in these basal organelles. However, some of the plastids localised in the rhizoids still contain DNA and those must play an active role during the process of regeneration (Puiseux-Dao and Dazy, 1970).

2. Autonomous functions of the plastids

(a) PHOTOSYNTHESIS

The photosynthetic activity of *Acetabularia* can of course be estimated by measuring oxygen evolution (Terborgh, 1966; Clauss, 1968) sometimes in a continual recording polarographic system, or else by measurements of the incorporation of radioactive $NaH^{14}CO_2$ (Clauss, 1968b). It depends essentially on the amount of light received, and the results are identical whether single or several algae (some of which inevitably afford shade to the others) are studied (Terborgh and McLeod, 1967). The wavelength of the light used is also very important. After a certain period of adaptation, continuous blue light (300 to 350 mμ) maintains a given level of photosynthesis (Fig. 37)

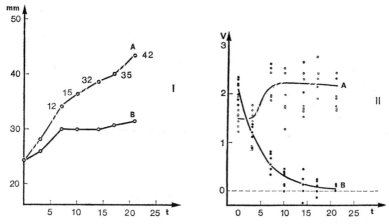

Figure 37. (I) Growth of *A. mediterranea* in blue light (A) or red light (B) of equivalent energy (4000 ergs cm^{-2}sec^{-1}). The numbers on the curves indicate the percentage of caps formed. *Abcissa*: time in days. *Ordinate*: the length of the algae in ml. (II) Photosynthetic activity of *A. mediterranea* (algae measuring 20 to 25 mm) in blue light (A) or red (B) light of equivalent energy (4000 ergs cm^{-2} sec^{-1}). *Abcissa*: time in days. *Ordinate*: the evolution of oxygen in µl per cell, for 2 hrs. (After Schael and Clauss, 1968.)

in both the *mediterranea* and the other species. On the other hand, constant red light of equal energy produces a more or less rapid fall in photosynthesis in *Acetabularia mediterranea* (Clauss, 1968, 1970); within three days, it is reduced by 40%, in seven days, to 70%, and at the end of two weeks has fallen to a negligible and undetectable level. When *Acetabularia crenulata* is illuminated with red light in the same way, photosynthetic activity falls to one third of its initial value by the end of forty-eight hours. Moreover, if the algae are cultured in red light for a sufficiently long period to arrest oxygen evolution, then transferred to blue light, photosynthesis is quickly stimulated (after a delay of only a few minutes in the case of *crenulata*, after several hours in the case of *mediterranea*). This renewal of photosynthesis occurs even if the duration of illumination with blue light is restricted to only a few seconds a day (thirty seconds for *Acetabularia mediterranea*, ten for the other). Short flashes of blue light interrupting constant red light also suffice to increase photosynthesis in the first species; the action of blue light is optimal at around 406–427 mµ in the first species, 450 mμ in the second. Inevitably, the effects of light wavelength reflect upon the development and morphogenesis of the algae, at least because of their influence on the synthesis of carbon chains and ATP (page 33).

It has been conclusively demonstrated in other plant materials easier to obtain in large quantities that the isolated plastids are capable of autonomous photosynthetic activity. Using plastids isolated from *Acetabularia*, Clauss (1968, 1969) found that red light does not permit photosynthesis, whereas with a normal light Shephard et al. (1968) observed gas evolution comparable to whole plants. These authors have further shown that the products of photosynthesis formed *in vitro* by the plastids are exactly the same as those formed *in vivo* by whole plants. Unfortunately, the plastids do not survive for very long, so their activity has been more especially studied, to date, in anucleate fragments of *Acetabularia*.

An analysis of the pigment content of the plastids in the anucleate fragments as compared with normal algae was undertaken by Richter (1958a). In the two experimental batches, chlorophylls were found as well as various carotenoids, mainly, in the order of their quantitative import-ance: lutein, β-carotene, neoxanthin, violaxanthin, and xantho-phyllepoxide. These pigments increase in quantity in a regular way during growth of whole algae. Similar measurements carried out with anucleate parts, whether basal or apical, indicate that a net synthesis of these pigments still takes place thirty days after enucleation, but the speed of synthesis of each of them is lower than in the nucleate fragments, which agrees with the observations made by Shephard (1965a), Zetsche (1969b) and Puiseux-Dao (1970) who arrived at the conclusion that the metabolism of the plastids is slower in *Acetabularia* deprived of a nucleus than in the controls.

Anucleate algae retain their photosynthetic capacities for more than four weeks, as has been shown from 1955 onwards by Brachet et al.; this finding confirms the great functional autonomy of the plastids. Isolated plastids are able to carry out photosynthesis (Shephard et al., 1968; Shephard, 1970). In any event, soluble sugars (fructose, saccharose, glucose and polymers of fructose) continue to be synthesised actively in the absence of the nucleus. They actually accumulate more than in normal

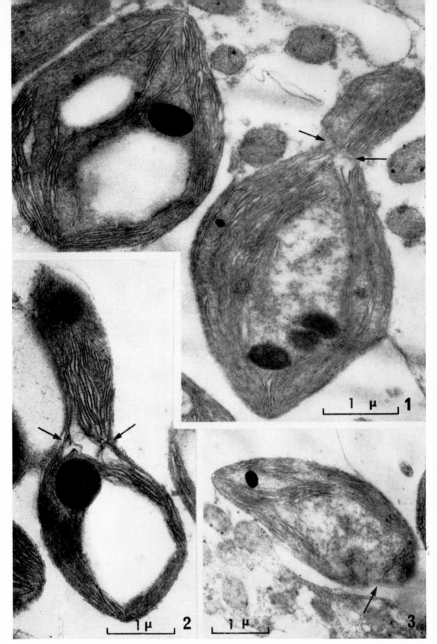

Plate 13. Division of the plastids in *A. mediterranea.* (1) Division of the peripheral saccules in a plastid undergoing division, observed in tangential section. (2) Beginning of the division of the peripheral saccules in a plastid about to divide. (3) Plastid presenting a sub-apical tear. The zone lacking a membrane is interpreted as the site of healing visible in the plastid after its division into two. (Ruseux-Dao, 1966 and unpublished.)

Acetabularia, probably because the carbon chains they supply are not used up in the anucleate fragments (Clauss and Keck, 1959). Abundant storage granules effectively appear in the plastids of anucleate fragments, making the study of their ultrastructure difficult but this accumulation appears as a consequence of the modes of nuclear control on plastid metabolism (Puiseux-Dao, 1970). Even after enucleation, the deleterious effects of red light are of course observed. Besides in whole algae, nuclear morphogenetic substances seem to be synthesised without inhibition, and are subsequently massed in the cytoplasm, just as they are when the algae are kept in the dark; they are used up only if the light source emits blue rays (Clauss, 1968).

The entirety of these results supports the view that the plastids of *Acetabularia* function in blue light, but lose their photosynthetic capacity in red light. The metabolism of these organelles influences the growth and morphogenesis of the whole algae. However, although the plastids in anucleate cytoplasm possess relatively long-lasting autonomy, their ability to synthesise normal pigments and sugars is sooner or later perturbed when exchanges are no longer possible between their cytoplasmic environment and the excised nucleus.

(b) PROTEIN SYNTHESIS AND RIBONUCLEIC ACID SYNTHESIS IN ISOLATED PLASTIDS

The prolonged survival of anucleate fragments of *Acetabularia* and especially the presence of DNA in the plastids, suggests that these organelles should be capable of synthesising, independently, a certain number of proteins.

High quantities of radioisotopes are incorporated when ^{14}C-aminoacids are added to the buffer solution, *pH* 6·9 containing mannitol, in which isolated chloroplasts from *Acetabularia* stalks are maintained. Analysis of the protein hydrolysate obtained from the plastids after experimentation by chromatography has demonstrated that incorporation effectively takes place into chloroplast proteins. Some of the amino acids, including leucine, iso-leucine, arginine, valine and phenylalanine are incorporated in higher quantities, all proportions maintained, than the others. Such labelling of the plastids with radioactive protein precursors is, moreover, inhibited strongly

9—AACB * *

by puromycin and actinomycin (Brachet and Goffeau, 1964; Goffeau and Brachet, 1965). These facts led to the conclusion that at least a fraction of the proteins synthesised in these organelles is monitored by the plastid DNA in an autonomous way, according to the traditional mechanism of genetic coding, using RNA as an intermediate. There is enough DNA in each plastid to allow it to code for several hundreds of proteins having a molecular weight of about 20,000 (Baltus and Brachet, 1963; Gibor and Izawa, 1963).

The synthesis of RNAs, notably of messenger RNAs, is necessarily implicated in protein synthesis coded for by DNA. Effectively, the isolated plastids supplied with ^{14}C-uracil *in vitro*, in buffer solution, incorporate this label by a mechanism which can be inhibited by actinomycin, by deoxyribonuclease and by maintenance in darkness (Schweiger and Berger, 1964). The addition to the medium, instead of uracil, of a mixture of the four nucleoside triphosphates (ATP, GTP, CTP, UTP) or of ATP labelled with ^{14}C, results in the appearance of radioactivity in an acid-soluble fraction which produces, by alkaline hydrolysis, the four 2 3 nucleoside phosphates (Schweiger and Berger, 1964; Brachet and Goffeau, 1964). However, this question is extremely complex (p. 71).*

These findings prove that in *Acetabularia* at least a part of the protein synthesis which takes place in the plastids is controlled by the DNA of these organelles, through the intermediate message carried by RNAs. However, after removal of the nucleus, such synthetic capacity fails to last longer than seven days in the basal parts, twenty-one to twenty-eight days in the apices, as the estimations made by Clauss seem to show (1958).

---

* Lipid analyses of whole *Acetabularia mediterranea* and plastid fractions give the following results: the most abundant fatty acids are palmitic acid (21% of fatty acids) and oleic acid (40%); phosphatidyl glycerol, phosphatidyl serine, phosphatidyl ethanolamine and phosphatidyl choline are present, as are mono- and digalactosyldiglycacids. The results approach those given for the few analysed green marine Algae, except for linolenic acid whose content is very low (Dubacq and Mazliake, unpublished).

B. THE PLASTID UNIT AND ITS REPLICATION

The chloroplasts of *Acetabularia* as seen with the electron microscope seem to be ovoid, more or less elongate organelles; they each contain one, two, three, sometimes more carbohydrate granules which can be stained brown with iodo-iodurate reagent, and which contain polymers of glucose and fructose (page 105). Maintenance of the *Acetabularia* in obscurity for more than a week results in a majority of elongate plastids containing three to eight carbohydrate granules (Puiseux-Dao and Dazy, 1970). Algae cultured in the presence of streptomycin contain only plastids with one single granule (Shephard, 1965a). This is also the case in the presence of ethidium bromide: the small forms predominate (Puiseux-Dao and Dazy, 1970). These observations led the authors to speculate on the possible existence of a fundamental morphological entity or basic unit which would contain only one single granule.

Now, studies of the ultrastructure of *Acetabularia mediterranea* plastids, and a careful analysis of the different facts revealed by the various pictures imposes the conclusion that the plastids divide according to a regular geometrical process which effectively results in the multiplication of a basic unit containing one carbohydrate granule (Puiseux-Dao, 1966). Serial longitudinal sections of small plastids containing one granule bring evidence of a simple structure which is approximately symmetrical about a slightly oblique longitudinal axis. This imaginary axis traverses the plastids from what can be designated as two opposite poles: P1 and P2. At each pole, groups of membranous ribbons folded upon themselves constitute stacked saccules surrounding the central granule. Most of the ribosomes, and the network of DNA possessed by these organelles, is situated between the carbohydrate granule and the lamellae. The whole organelle is enclosed in a double membrane (page 44 and Fig. 39). Serial sections have confirmed a similar organisation in chloroplasts with two granules. One special feature emerges: the two granules are always separated by lamellae which are attached to the two opposite poles. These internal lamellae which can conveniently be called the 'diagonal' lamellae because of their arrangement, each seem preferentially to surround the carbohydrate granule nearest the pole to which they are attached. Each sub-unit made up of a granule and surrounding saccules therefore resembles a whole plastid with one carbohydrate storage granule. Functionally, the double structure would allow the formation of two daughter plastids each possessing one carbohydrate granule by a kind of tangential sliding, with regard to the two groups of lamellae (Fig. 38). In this case, a certain number of plastids containing one granule would be expected to be slightly torn away near to one of the poles, at the point at which the plastid envelope and subjacent saccules have come apart. Such rupture points are effectively often observed (Plate 13). The healing of this zone might be thought to be easy, given the facility of morphogenesis of the plastid membranes. However, one finding remains to be elucidated: the formation of the second carbohydrate granule and of diagonal lamellae in chloroplasts containing only one granule. Careful observation of sections near to the central axis in the apical zone reveals a certain assymmetry, one side of some of the sectioned plastids bearing more lamellae than the other; among these lamellae, a small field of stroma occurs. It seems logical to infer that this zone is equivalent to a sec-ond carbohydrate centre under formation, separated from the first by a number of diagonal plastid membranes. These findings and their explanation leads us to propose a simple diagram of plastid structure in *Acetabularia mediterranea* (Fig. 39).

This picture is, however, somewhat simplified, and the facts are more complex. Plastids containing one and two granules are not the only ones which exist in *Acetabularia*; chloroplasts containing three or more carbohydrate centres are also encountered. In chloroplasts of the upper part of the algae, electron microscopy never fails to reveal separating ribbons of diagonally arranged lamellae between each storage grain; each granule is thus surrounded by membranous tongues diverging from the two diametrically opposite poles. The plastids having only one granule therefore correspond to a basic morphological entity. The replication of this basic unit would sometimes be more rapid than the dissociation of the resulting new elements, as is sometimes the case during bacterial division, and would

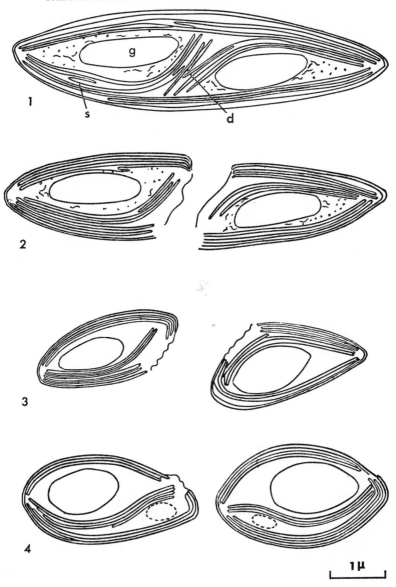

Figure 38. Diagram of the division of the plastids in *Acetabularia* (Puiseux-Dao, 1970). (1) Plastids with 2 units. (2) Subdivision of the 2 units by the cutting through of the external saccules. (3) Healing of the daughter plastids. (4) Growth of the daughter plastids and formation of a second unit in each of them, that is to say, either near to the zone of healing (left) or on the opposite side (right).

therefore lead, in this case, to the formation of big chloroplasts containing several grains, more numerous when growth of the alga is slow.

In algae kept in the dark (Puiseux-Dao and Dazy, 1970) it should be mentioned that the chloroplasts are found to be very long, and they cannot be stained with the iodo-iodurate reagent although, under the culture conditions used, they retain storage granules for a prolonged period of up to several weeks, which are visible under the electron microscope. Up to eight grains per chloroplast could be counted under the culture conditions (Plate 10). The occasional L form of some of the plastids suggests that some of them have fused together, as Shephard (1965a) thought on the basis of his own optical observations. When the algae are kept in the dark for eight to fifteen days, the peripheral lamellar structure in such giant plastids is deficient or arranged abnormally in stacked piles of short saccules; the diagonal lamellae still exist, however. Logically, it may be assumed that these are chloroplasts composed of six, seven or eight units, which separate progressively from one another when the algae are returned to the light (Plate 10).

The structural diagram which is proposed concerning the plastids of *Acetabularia* and their mode of division, raises the problem of DNA replication and the separation of the fibres of this molecule in such a way that each daughter unit receives a supply of DNA. The most economical hypothesis would seem to involve the drawing of half the DNA along the length of one of the diagonal lamellae, which would thus act as a guiding track, as suggested by the diagram (Fig. 39). The plastids of *Acetabularia mediterranea* would, in this event, be composed of three different kinds of membrane: those of the external envelope, those of the photosynthetic saccules and those of the

---

Figure 39. (1) Diagram of the arrangement of the saccules in an *Acetabularia* plastid having one carbohydrate granule. (2) to (5) Diagram of the hypothesis concerning the existence of three kinds of lamellae in *Acetabularia* plastids. (A) external plastid membrane; (B) photosynthetic saccules (more or less developed); (C) diagonal lamellae associated with DNA, symbolised by black dots. The carbohydrate granule of each unit has been drawn, for the sake of the diagram, as if it were attached to the corresponding stock of DNA. (2) Plastids having 2 units. (3) Division of the plastids. (4) and (4A) Formation of a second unit in the plastids and daughter. (Puiseux-Dao, unpublished.)

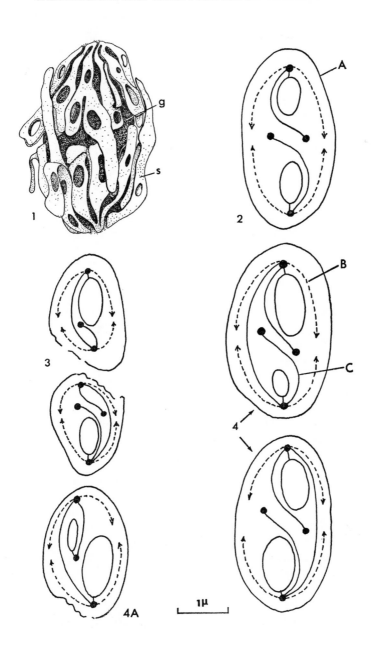

diagonal lamellae carrying the DNA in contact with the internal stroma. This seems to fit in very well with the behaviour observed in plastids kept in the dark: under these circumstances the envelope always persists, the diagonal lamellae always remain in place between the carbohydrate granules, but within the first few days in the dark and, especially after about fifteen days, the peripheral saccules are very rapidly reduced in length and appear stacks of short disks; they are thus extremely susceptible to the absence of light (Puiseux-Dao and Dazy, 1970).

This idea seems very feasible, that the plastids of *Acetabularia* are made up of one or several identical units, each of which is able to replicate. The number of units which remain associated together depends essentially on the general conditions of culture; in the presence of streptomycin or ethidium bromide, only single basic units usually occur, probably because their separation has taken place, but not their replication, which would be blocked by these substances. Conversely, in the dark, the plastids would form relatively long chains of several units for quite opposite reasons. In basal plastids, the study of these units of structure and of their evolution remains difficult, except when severed basal rhizoids are allowed to regenerate. It should be added that the diagram advanced to explain the situation in *Acetabularia mediterranea* seems to be equally valid for other species, judging from electron microscope observations on *Acetabularia peniculus, killneri* and *clavata* (Puiseux-Dao, unpublished).

C. THE FUNCTIONAL PERIODICITY OF THE PLASTIDS

Most living cells have rhythmic activity related to the alternation of day and night; in fact, even under constant light conditions, the functional rhythm of some of these organelles persists for a fairly long time: such cases are defined as examples of 'endogenous rhythm'. In plants, *a priori*, photosynthetic activity must be rhythmically related to light, and this phenomenon has naturally attracted investigation, especially in *Acetabularia*.

1. Circadian rhythms and plastid activity

Sweeney and Haxo undertook in 1961 to study the photosynthetic rhythm of *Acetabularia crenulata* and *Acetabularia major*. Measurements were made at midday and at midnight on algae which, after having been kept in natural light conditions, were maintained for an experimental period in constant low light (30 ft-ca) or in total darkness; the temperature and the composition of the medium were of course kept constant. Photosynthetic activity was estimated after thirty minutes adaptation to saturating light intensities of 1,500 ft-ca by measurement of the amount of oxygen liberated per hour and per unit fresh weight: striking periodicity was observed (Fig. 40). Alternating high and low values of gas evolution were recorded at midday and at midnight respectively, exactly as in algae placed in normal light conditions; the endogenous rhythm is maintained for several days. Very sudden change in the photoperiodicity of external light supply, involving complete reversal of phase, results on the contrary in concomitant inversion of photosynthetic period, in adaptation to the new situation (Fig. 40). Identical results were recorded with *Acetabularia mediterranea*, using measurements of oxygen evolution by a new electrochemical technique (Schweiger et al., 1964; von Klitzing and Schweiger, 1968). The duration of the light period, in these experiments, was twelve hours (12L—12D) and the amount of oxygen evolved per plant and per hour followed a rhythm which, once again, was maintained by such algae when they were transferred to constant light. Rhythm was maintained for a long period, since it was still observed after three weeks. The reversal of light periodicity results in an inversion of rhythm. Terborgh and McLeod (1967) were able to confirm these findings with *Acetabularia crenulata*; they studied continuous instead of intermittent measurements of oxygen evolution, using a polarographic apparatus equipped with a graphite cathode. Bimodal curves were obtained. They show that in normal light a dramatic increase in oxygen evolution occurs when the light is *put on* (stage 1); subsequently, a drop occurs which lasts about thirty minutes, followed again by an increase beginning about one hour after illumination has started. At the end of approximately three hours the initial maximum is largely

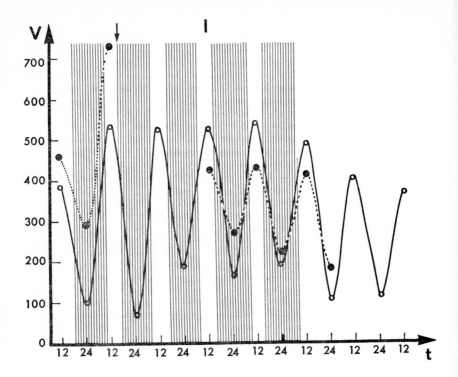

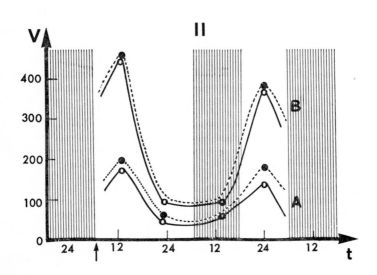

exceeded (stage 2) and the slope becomes much more gentle (Fig. 41). The fall in oxygen evolution when the light is *put off* is exceedingly rapid, so that the nocturnal level is reached within thirty minutes. Graphic recordings of a similar nature have been achieved in permanent light of variable intensity, either approaching a saturation level (1,000 ft-ca) or below this (250 ft-ca and 45 ft-ca). In all three situations rhythm is maintained, but a slight shift in the oscillations as compared with the normal tends to suggest that the period of endogenous rhythm slightly exceeds twenty-four hours (about twenty-five hours). It suffices to illuminate only once according to the normal day/night alternation to restore the corresponding diurnal/nocturnal oscillation.

All these measurements of oxygen evolution provide evidence of *circadian rhythm* affecting photosynthesis, at least as far as light reactions are concerned. The same endogenous activity governs the incorporation of $^{14}CO_2$ ($NaH^{14}CO_3$) in *Acetabularia crenulata* (Richter, 1963; Hellebust et al., 1967); the dark reactions are thus under the control of oscillations of a circadian type.

The question is thus raised whether pigments and catalytic enzymes involved in photosynthesis are also synthesised according to a similar rhythm. The total content of chlorophyll seemed to vary according to the photoperiod imposed upon the alga (page 116) and the question therefore seemed important. However, estimations of chlorophyll content have provided a negative answer to this query (Hellebust et al., 1967). The

---

Figure 40. Rhythm of photosynthetic activity in *A. major*. (I) The algae were kept in normal light for the 1st 5 days of the experiment, then placed in constant light (30 ft-ca). Photosynthetic activity (average based on measurements made on 10 young algae without caps (broken line) or an algae with a cap (continuous line) after 30 mins illumination in saturating light (1500 ft-ca) at 25°C). The algae were anucleated after the first measurements (arrow). (II) Adaptation of the rhythm of photosynthetic activity in *A. crenulata*. Normal algae (continuous line) and anucleate fragments (broken line) have been kept under the conditions described above (I), then subjected to an inversion of light rhythm by the interposition of a light period double the normal length. The maximum of photosynthetic activity is displayed during the first light period which follows; it always occurs in the middle of this period. (A) Photosynthetic activity (average) of 5 young algae. (B) Average photosynthetic activity of an alga with a cap. *Abcissa*: time in days (nights by diagonal hatching). *Ordinate*: quantity of oxygen (v) evolved per hr and per g of fresh wt (wet wt). (After Sweeney and Haxo, 1961).

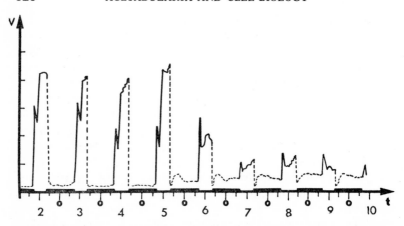

Figure 41. Evolution of oxygen exchange in *A. crenulata*. Light cycle: 8 hrs of
light (250 ft-ca) and 16 hrs of dark (o). Temperature: 28°C. From the fifth day
onwards, a fall in the exchange, thought to be due to the direct toxic effect of the
electrode. *Abcissa*: time in days. *Ordinate*: evolution of oxygen in arbitrary units.
(After Terborgh and McLeod, 1967.)

enzymes of the pentose pathway, notably ribulose-1-5-diphos-
phate carboxylase have also been studied. No difference was
observed between algae examined during the light as compared
with the dark periods. The presence and activity of eight other
enzymes was also found to be constant: the activity of five of
them: phosphoglycerate kinase; D-glyceraldehyde-3-phosphate
dehydrogenase, triosephosphate isomerase, ribose-5-phosphate
isomerase and ribulose-6-phosphate kinase, are much higher
than is required for saturation level incorporation of CO_2,
whereas the three others: aldolase, transketolase and transaldo-
lase and the ribulose 1-5 diphosphate carboxylase are found in
amounts which correspond to the speed of assimilation of CO_2
at saturation light levels (Hellebust et al., 1967).

Since photosynthesis culminates in the formation of carbon
chains which are stored mainly as fructosans in the Dasycladales, estimations of these sugars have been carried out on
pellets of isolated plastids at various intervals throughout the
light cycle. The quantity of fructosans detected in the isolated
plastids varies considerably throughout the day in *Acetabularia
mediterranea*. The level is low in the early morning, equivalent
to only 25 μg; it rises to 65 μg at the end of the afternoon. This

variation is rhythmic and persists in continuous light, thus showing its endogenous character (Vanden Driessche and Bonotto, 1968a). Synthesis of ATP also shows a rhythmic activity (von Klitzing, 1969; Vanden Driessche, 1970). Cytoplasmic RNA synthesis also seems to be subjected to a circadian rhythm, as shown by studies of ^{3}H-uridine incorporation into acid-insoluble fraction from *Acetabularia* cells; the RNAs concerned are probably chloroplastic (Vanden Driessche and Bonotto, 1968b, 1969; Vanden Driessche, 1970) but this rhythm allows special features.

The morphology of the chloroplasts evolves according to circadian rhythm, just like their physiological behaviour. Indeed, Vanden Driessche (1966a) discovered that in *Acetabularia* these organelles are much longer during the light period than during the dark period; for this reason, she measured the long and short axes of the plastids, under different light conditions. All the measurements were confined to the stalk in the region of the last whorl, where the transparency of the thin membrane makes observation much easier. Most of these observations were carried out with the aid of photographic enlargements of light microscopy, concerning the dimensions of the plastids (only the plastids exceeding a certain size were measured). In the middle of the light period, the plastids were found to be longer than in the dark. The ratio between the lengths of the two axes passes from 2·59 to 5·54 (Figs. 42 and 43) whereas the concomitant increase in oxygen evolution is 5. In order to ensure that measurements made with the light microscope were not distorted because of plastid movement, sections tangential to or perpendicular to the axis of the stalk were examined with the electron microscope: this analysis confirmed the previous findings. Alternating changes in chloroplast size follow the same periodicity when the algae are transferred to constant light. Periodic oscillations in photosynthesis and in the shape of the plastids are quite clearly correlated at all times (Vanden Driessche, 1966b). But the circadian rhythms are labile and liable to be lost, under certain circumstances, notably when the algae remain two weeks in the dark. The arhythmic *Acetabularia* so obtained recuperate their cyclic period as soon as they are subjected once again to alternate light and darkness (Vanden Driessche, 1966a).

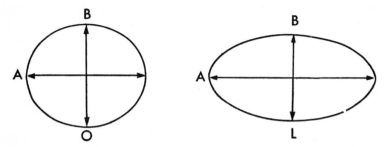

Figure 42. Diagram of the rhythmic variations in the shape of the plastids in *A. mediterranea*. (O) middle of the dark period; (L) middle of the light period; (A) long axis of the plastid; (B) short axis. (After Vanden Driessche, 1967b.)

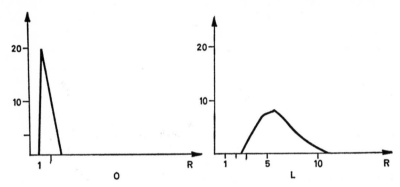

Figure 43. Distribution of the ratio (R) of the axis of the plastids in *A. mediterranea*. (O) middle of the dark period; (L) middle of the light period. (After Vanden Driessche, 1967b.)

2. The rhythm of multiplication of the plastids

Apart from their physiology and their shape, chloroplast multiplication may also evolve rhythmically. If the idea of plastid units described above is correct, it is relatively easy to find out how many units each plastid possesses by counting the number of carbohydrate granules present in them, after staining with the iodo-iodurate reagent. Counts of this kind have been performed in the following way on *Acetabularia mediterranea*: the contents of the upper two-thirds of the algal stalk are squeezed out on to glass slides and examined with the light microscope. The algae examined were obtained from cultures illuminated at 1,200 lux (light/dark periods of 11/13 hours respectively); light was administered from about seven o'clock in the morning onwards. Plastids having one, two, three and more granules were counted in populations of several hundreds of plastids for each hour of the day, from nine to eighteen hours. Plastids having only one granule were in the majority (55%) in the morning, whereas plastids containing at least three granules (P_3) were relatively infrequent at that time (10%). The number of plastids containing two granules hardly varies at all throughout the day. A steady increase in the number of plastids containing three or more granules is recorded as the day advances, whereas the percentage of small ones diminishes, gradually. The proportions then became: 23% (P_1), 54% (P_2), 25% (P_3). From five o'clock (17h) onwards the reverse takes place and values approaching those of the morning are gradually attained (Fig. 44). These findings can be interpreted in the following way: during the morning, new units are formed; about half the plastids having one grain (these are the most numerous) give rise to plastids containing two granules; roughly half the plastids with two granules develop a third. After seventeen hours, the separation of the newly formed plastid units is the dominant activity, so that some of the P_2 and P_3 plastids lose one unit, and a net increase in the number of small chloroplasts occurs. This daily fluctuation in plastid population is obviously rhythmic, whether endogenously so, or otherwise, was not verified. However, as has already been mentioned, after eight days in the dark, many of the plastids are elongate and fusions have probably occurred. The carbohydrate stores they contain are no longer stainable with the iodo-iodurate reagent, but become so after only one hour's illumination. Counts which are then performed on such algae replaced under normal light conditions show the loss in rhythm previously described, and do not regain it before a lapse of four to five days (Puiseux-Dao and Gilbert, 1967). Analogous results have been obtained after keeping algae in the dark for two to seven weeks. Percentage findings, although scarcely analysed as yet, suggest that under these circumstances, the normal periodicity affecting the formation and separation of new units is masked by the isolation of units which had fused together in the absence of light.

This regular process of formation of new units succeeded by

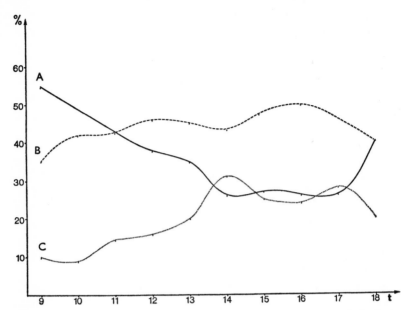

Figure 44. Distribution of the plastids possessing 1, 2 or more carbohydrate granules in *A. mediterranea* during the day (light: 1200 lux for 7 to 18 hr; temperature: 18°C). *Abcissa*: time in hours. *Ordinate*: percentage of plastids with 1 granule (A), 2 granules (B) and 3 or more granules (C). (After Puiseux-Dao and Gilbert, 1967.)

their subdivision into structures containing one granule, culminates finally in a progressive increase in the cell population of plastids. Enough numerical findings are now available with percentages and their variations, to be able to establish a mathematical law controlling the growth of this population; it is exponential, and can be expressed by the following formula:

$$Q_n = Q_0 \left(1 + \frac{\Delta x_0 + \Delta y_0}{x_0 + 2y_0 + 3z_0} \right)^n$$

Q_0 and Q_n are the number of plastids produced on the first and the nth day respectively; x_0, y_0 and z_0 are the percentages of plastids containing one, two and three or more granules in the morning; Δx_0 and Δy_0 corresponding to the maximum decrease in the percentage of plastids containing one and two granules during the day; n is the number of days (Puiseux-Dao, 1968).

The ratio $\dfrac{\Delta x_o + \Delta y_o}{x_o + 2y_o + 3z_o}$ is an experimental constant for a given culture; the law is exponential, in agreement with the measurements made by Shephard (1965). This law defines the growth of the plastid population, which is more rapid when the number of newly formed units is greater and slower when separation of new units is infrequent so that the big plastids predominate. The calculations show that under culture conditions, where one most frequently has $x_o = 55$, $y_o = 35$, $z_o = 10$, $\Delta x_o = 25$ and $\Delta y_o = 10$, the number of chloroplasts doubles in five days (Puiseux Dao, 1968). By counting, Shephard (1965a) evaluated the time required for the population to double as seven days, in slightly different culture conditions. Given that, in calculations, the plastids having more than three units have been disregarded, whereas they actually symbolise a slowing down in population growth, and so have the cyclotic movements which more or less alter the distribution of these organelles, the agreement between calculation and measurements is fairly good. This agreement seems to support the idea of basic plastid units in *Acetabularia*.

It seems worth while emphasising that the genesis of new units following the process previously described implies a diurnal lengthening of certain plastids and, conversely, nocturnal shortening, which is not incompatible with the measurements made by Vanden Driessche (1966b). The modifications this author describes must embody this phenomenon, which overlies the changes in shape proper to the plastids themselves.

3. Nuclear control of circadian rhythm

Early on, *Acetabularia* was used for the study of the role of the nucleus in the maintenance of circadian rhythms and in 1961, Sweeney and Haxo, after noticing that cutting the alga in two halves had but little effect on photosynthesis in adult plants, whereas the opposite is true for young *Acetabularia* (*A. major* and *A. crenulata*), went on to indicate that enucleation has no effect on the endogenous rhythm affecting photosynthetic activity. This is also the case in the *mediterranea* species, forty to fifty days after the amputation of the nucleate half (Richter, 1963; Schweiger et al., 1964a). Moreover, Vanden

10—AACB

Driessche was able to show (1966) that in the latter species not only the photosynthetic rhythm, but also the oscillating changes affecting the shape of the plastids, remain unaffected by enucleation. Further, when the rhythm of the anucleate fragments is destroyed by a two weeks' stay in the dark, it is nevertheless recovered when the fragments are brought back into the light.

The problem of nuclear control of circadian rhythm in *Acetabularia* remains a difficult one, however, since nuclear interference in the cytoplasm of these big cells is characterised by remarkable stability and autonomy. Experimental grafting and nuclear implantations have enabled Schweiger et al. (1964b) to demonstrate that, taking into account the difficulty of experimental conditions, the nucleus can be considered to impose its own phase on the cytoplasm. After having induced opposite phases in two batches of *Acetabularia*, insofar as photosynthetic rhythm is concerned, they performed uninucleate grafts involving a basal nucleate part having one phase, and an anucleate stalk adapted to a second phase. The algae so obtained are dominated by the rhythm belonging to the nucleate half (Fig. 45). The same authors used perforated shields against the light in order to illuminate stalks and rhizoids of the same algae in phase opposition: here again, measurements of oxygen evolution confirmed that the intact cells tended to acquire the rhythm induced by external light on the *nuclear* part. Two graft combinations between algae with and without photosynthetic rhythm have been achieved by Vanden Driessche (1967a) with results which confirm that external light induces photosynthetic rhythmicity at the level of the nucleus. The photosynthetic rhythmicity is accompanied by an oscillation of the ATP cell content (Vanden Driessche, 1970).

To the same end, Vanden Driessche (1966) has treated whole algae with actinomycin D. This substance very strongly inhibited the periodicity affecting photosynthetic activity; the intensity of effect was proportional to the concentration used. Striking reduction in photosynthetic rhythm was achieved after six days treatment with 2·7 μg actinomycin/ml; about twelve days at least are required to produce the same effect when the concentration is reduced tenfold. Variations in chloroplast shape are concomitantly eliminated. Yet actinomycin D has no

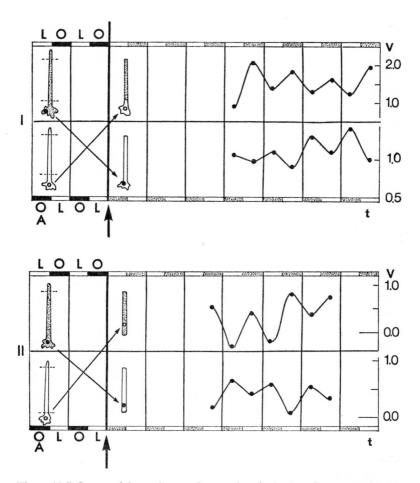

Figure 45. Influence of the nucleus on the cytoplasmic rhythm of oxygen exchange in *A. mediterranea*. (I) Transplantation of the rhizoids. The rhizoids and the anucleate fragments derived from algae displaying opposite rhythm. After grafting, the algae were placed in constant light. (II) Implantation of nuclei under the same conditions as (I). *Abcissa*: time in days. *Ordinate*: the evolution of oxygen in μl per plant and per hr. (Schweiger et al., 1964a.)

effect on the circadian rhythms affecting photosynthesis in the *anucleate* fragments, whether they are basal or apical. The implication of these findings is that only nuclear (and not cytoplasmic) DNA is involved in controlling the biological clock, and that its action requires the intermediate functioning of relatively long lived messenger RNAs able to remain stable in the anucleate stalks; the latter, or the molecules they have induced, certainly survive longer in anucleate fragments than in controls, since the rhythm persists several weeks in the absence of the nucleus, whereas in nucleate algae the effects of actinomycin make themselves felt after several days only.

Since circadian rhythms of the plastids differ from morphogenetic capacity in that no functional difference distinguishes basal anucleate from apical fragments, it seems plausible to imagine that inside the cytoplasm nuclear messages on this subject are uniformly distributed, perhaps in the form of complexes (Vanden Driessche, 1966b, 1967a).

However, the intervention of RNAs coming from the nucleus is not easy to elucidate. Photosynthetic capacity drops, but its rhythm persists in whole algae treated with 1 mg ribonuclease per ml, for eight days. When, after a week or more, the algae are replaced in a normal medium, photosynthetic activity and the degree of periodicity increase considerably as compared with the controls. The dry weight of the plants simultaneously diminishes, probably because of the action of the enzyme, since even after eight days restoration of normal conditions, it is lower than that of controls (15·5 mg for 25 algae instead of 17·3 mg). Subsequently, the dry weight rises above normal after several weeks (24·5 mg for 15 treated algae, as compared with 18·6 mg for controls). It is interesting to compare these findings (Vanden Driessche, 1966b) with the results already described concerning the action of ribonuclease (page 87) which indicates a net depression of cytoplasmic activity in the presence of the enzyme, followed by a secondary stimulatory effect probably due to the increased emission of nuclear messages. Restoration of photosynthetic rhythm after ribonuclease treatment is not possible in the absence of the nucleus (Vanden Driessche, 1966b). Chloramphenicol, tested as an inhibitor of the translation of the genetic code, rapidly destroys (48h) circadian rhythm in *Acetabularia*, which implicates protein synthesis in the maintenance of this process (Vanden Driessche, 1967b). Rifampicin, a specific inhibitor of transcription in chloroplasts and mitochondria has no effect on the rhythms in photosynthesis, a finding which also suggests the existence of a control outside the plastids (Vanden Driessche, 1970).

The various results obtained in this field suggest that plastid DNA directly controls some syntheses, involving fairly rapid turnover of a part at least of lamellar structures as well as of a variable proportion of the plastidal enzymes; the immediate effect of ribonuclease and chloramphenicol and the slower effect of actinomycin on the morphology of the thylacoids and on photosynthetic activity are not incompatible with such an interpretation. On the other hand the nucleus directly controls, among other plastidal functions, the circadian rhythms; this control must involve protein intermediates elaborated with the aid of one or more nuclear messenger RNAs, since chloramphenicol alone produces a rapid effect, unlike ribonuclease and contrary, *a fortiori*, to actinomycin.

Thus, the plastids of *Acetabularia* are relatively independent organelles. Their autonomy depends on the one hand on the presence of intrinsic DNA able to code for the synthesis of several hundreds of proteins, and probably most especially for those proteins which are required for the replication of this DNA itself, and for transmitting its orders. However, the average length of life of nuclear messages is from ten to fifteen days in these algae, and their persistence is able to ensure a phase of autonomy to the plastids of the anucleate fragments. The photosynthetic activity of these organelles is subject to circadian rhythm, itself correlated with periodic, endogenous changes in chloroplast shape. Rhythmic oscillations are also typical of the multiplication of the plastids, which follows an exponential law. Endogenous rhythms are under nuclear control: their study is one of the research pathways which can lead to a better understanding of the interrelations between the nucleus and the organelles containing satellite DNA. Present knowledge suggests that at least two mechanisms exist whereby the nucleus exerts control over the plastids (Puiseux-Dao, 1970).

7

Conclusions

Acetabularia are certainly the best known of the marine algae, a few species of which have been cultured in large quantities for laboratory purposes. In spite of the disadvantage which resides in their slow rate of growth, they have attracted research aiming, in general, at one main purpose, that of piercing the secret of cell life. For the morphologist, what great satisfaction there is to be obtained from the analysis of the manifold morphogenetic possibilities of these giant cells, culminating in the creation of a very complete, very complicated and at the same time very beautiful achievement of nature! Systematic and ecological work suggests that the repertoire of the smaller species is still incomplete. Among the numerous *Acetabularia* recently discovered, there may be laboratory materials more convenient for experimental purposes than those usually studied. But it must be said that the domestication of *Acetabularia* is not an easy task, and perhaps it is for this reason that in general, investigators tend to pursue their research with the species which circulate at present, among the different laboratories. There are two main reasons for this state of affairs: the problem of sterility is more acute with algae coming from nature; moreover, families which develop rapidly and have a shorter period of dormancy have finally been selected by the different research groups. Culture conditions, however, have gradually, though slowly, been improved. Various aspects, such as the light requirements of the algae, are better known. The complexity of the culture medium required by the algae is a complicating factor which excludes the achievement of certain experiments of a physiological nature. Further, the duration of development which, at best, lasts several months, implies the constant and time-taking maintenance of the cultures.

In spite of all these disadvantages, no other biological material has proved so useful for the study of nucleocytoplasmic relationships in Eukaryotes. The ease with which nucleate and anucleate fragments can be obtained has resulted in the success of a great deal of significant biological work. Cytological study of this material immediately showed that these cells possess three main centres of activity: the nucleus, the apical zone of morphogenesis and the chloroplasts. The nucleus, which is very probably polyploid, is large and contains a basophilic nuclear mass which is extremely sensitive towards metabolic variations to which the cells are submitted: amputation of a part of the cytoplasm, presence of inhibitors in the medium, action of radiations. All these results, as observed in the light and the electron microscope, prove that the nucleus is a centre rich in RNAs and in proteins, a high proportion of which would constitute the ribosomes. Autoradiographic and biochemical investigations always lead to the same conclusion. In agreement with cytological findings, they confirm the existence of a dynamic factor, the movement of ribonucleoprotein complexes from the nucleus into the cytoplasm (the complexes being formed either before or after leaving the nucleus). In the algal stalk these substances of nuclear origin, according to autoradiographic and metabolic studies, seem to fall into two categories: most of them are concentrated in the apical zone of morphogenesis; a few are uniformly distributed throughout the cytoplasm. In every case, experimental associations of all kinds, including grafts, the use of specific inhibitors acting on nucleate and anucleate fragments, have brought evidence of the fact that the substances of nuclear origin containing the specific messages are fairly long-lived. The messages which accumulate in the apices, where they are responsible for morphogenesis, probably take the form of polysomes. Among those which are emitted simultaneously at a given time, some are translated instantaneously by the cytoplasm, others are only used to code for proteins later on; the reading of nuclear messages is regulated in the cytoplasm itself. An ordered synthesis, particularly of proteins, and of enzymes, seems to be indispensable for normal morphogenesis, not only of the axial stalk with its sterile whorls, but also for the creation of a reproductive cap. The completion of the upright stalk, then of the cap, takes place in two stages which, if they occur consecutively without rupture of the curve of development, are associated with progressive changes in the biochemical components of the cell.

Other nuclear messages disseminated throughout the cytoplasm probably concern the plastids and doubtless, also, the mitochondria. The former of these organelles elaborates carbon chains, a certain number of proteins, pigments and ATP. Their metabolism, like that of the nucleus, is readily disturbed by experimental factors the effects of which are often visible on an ultrastructural level. The activity of these organelles, which are capable of multiplying themselves, shows functional periodicity bound to a nycthermeral rhythm of endogenous nature, placed under nuclear control, and effectuated without any doubt through the intermediary of the messages mentioned above.

The sum of all the results obtained with *Acetabularia* form an elaborate yet coherent whole of considerable significance with regard to nucleocytoplasmic relationships. With patient analysis, the knowledge acquired will make it possible to extricate from a tangle of facts, the basic rules underlying cell mechanisms: the specialised functioning of each of the types of cell organelles, the coordination of their function to the greater benefit of the cell as a whole, the nuclear control of the intracellular balance required for specific and normal morphology, as well as the specific cell function which consists in the conservation, at genetic level, of the cell potential, whether this genetic potential be expressed or not.

REFERENCES

ATTARDI, G., PARNAS, H., HWANG, M. I. and ATTARDI, B. (1966) Giant-size rapidly labelled Nuclear Ribonucleic Acid and Cytoplasmic Messenger Ribonucleic Acid in Immature Duck Erythrocytes. *J. Mol. Biol.* **21**, 145–182.

BACQ, Z. M., VANDERHAEGHE, F., DAMBLON, J., ERRERA, M. and HERVE, A. (1957) Effets des rayons X sur *Acetabularia mediterranea. Exptl. Cell Res.* **12**, 639–648.

BALTUS, E. (1959) Evolution de l'aldolase dans les fragments anucléés d'*Acetabularia. Bioch. Bioph. Acta.* **33**, 337–339.

BALTUS, E. and BRACHET, J. (1962) Le dosage de l'Acide Désoxyribonucléique dans les oeufs de Batraciens. *Bioch. Bioph. Acta* **61**, 1957–163.

BALTUS, E. and BRACHET, J. (1963) Presence of deoxyribonucleic Acid in the Chloroplast of *Acetabularia mediterranea. Bioch. Bioph. Acta* **76**, 490–492.

BALTUS, E., EDSTRÖM, J. E., JANOWSKI, M., HANOCQ-QUERTIER, J., TENCER, R. and BRACHET, J. (1968) Base Composition and Metabolism of Various RNA-Fractions in *Acetabularia mediterranea. Proc. Nat. Acad. Sci.* **59**, 406–413.

BALTUS, E. and QUERTIER, J. (1966) A Method for the Extraction and Characterization of RNA from subcellular Fractions of *Acetabularia. Bioch. Bioph. Acta* **119**, 192–194.

BARY, A. de and STRASBURGER, E. (1877) *Acetabularia mediterranea. Bot. Ztg.* **35**, 713–755.

BERGER, S. (1967) RNA-Synthesis in *Acetabularia.* II. RNA-synthesis in isolated chloroplasts. *Protoplasma* **64**, 13–25.

BERKALOFF, C. (1967) Modifications ultrastructurales du plaste et de divers autres organites cellulaires au cours du développement et de l'enkystement du *Protosyphon botryoides* (Chlorophycées). *J. Microsc.* **6**, 839–852.

BETH, K. (1943a) Entwicklung und Regeneration von *Acetabularia Schenckii. Ztg. Abstamm. u. Vererbungslehre* **81**, 252–270.

BETH, K. (1943b) Ein- und zweikernige Transplantate zwischen *Acetabularia mediterranea* und *Acicularia Schenckii. Ztg. Abstamm. u. Vererbungslehre* **81**, 271–312.

BETH, K. (1943c) Ein- und zweikernige Transplantate verschiedener Acetabulariaceen. *Naturwissenschaften* **31**, 206–207.

BETH, K. (1953a) Experimentelle Untersuchungen über die Wirkung des Lichtes auf die Formbildung von kernhaltigen und kernlosen *Acetabularia* Zellen. *Z. Naturforsch.* **8b**, 334–342.

BETH, K. (1953b) Ueber den Einfluss des Kernes auf die Formbildung von *Acetabularia* in verschiedenen Entwicklungstadien. *Z. Naturforsch.* **8b**, 771–775.

BETH, K. (1955a) Beziehungen zwischen Wachstum und Formbildung in Abhängigkeit von Licht und Temperatur bei *Acetabularia. Z. Naturforsch.* **10b**, 267–276.

BETH, K. (1955b) Unterschiedliche Beeinflussung von Wachstum und

Teilung durch Veränderung von Licht und Temperatur. *Z. Natur-forsch.* **10b**, 276–281.

BOLOUKHÈRE-PRESBURG, M. (1965) Effets de l'actinomycine D sur l'ultra-structure des chloroplastes et du noyau d'*Acetabularia mediterranea*. *J. Microsc.* **4**, 363–372.

BOLOUKHÈRE-PRESBURG, M. (1966) Effets de la puromycine sur l'ultra-structure d'*Acetabularia mediterranea*. *J. Microsc.* **5**, 619–628.

BOLOUKHÈRE-PRESBURG, M. (1969) Ultrastructure de l'Algue *Acetabularia mediterranea* au cours du cycle biologique et dans différentes conditions expérimentales. Thèse, Université libre de Bruxelles.

BOLOUKHÈRE-PRESBURG, M. (1970) Ultrastructure of *Acetabularia mediterranea* in the course of the formation of secondary nuclei. In *Biology of Acetabularia*. Edrs. Brachet, J. and Bonotto, S. Academic Press, New York and London, 145–176.

BONOTTO, S. (1968) Sur la formation de chapeaux anormaux chez *Acetabularia mediterranea*. *Protoplasma* **66**, 55–61.

BONOTTO, S. (1970) Effects of gamma-radiation on *Acetabularia mediterranea*. In *Biology of Acetabularia*. Edrs. Brachet, J. and Bonotto, S. Academic Press, New York and London, 255–272.

BONOTTO, S., GOFFEAU, A., JANOWSKI, M., VANDEN DRIESSCHE, T. and BRACHET, J. (1969) Effects of various inhibitors of protein synthesis on *Acetabularia mediterranea*. *Bioch. Bioph. Acta* **174**, 704–712.

BONOTTO, S. and JANOWSKI, M. (1968) Dichotomie du siphon chez *Acetabularia mediterranea*. *Bull. Acad. Roy. belg.* **54**, 1369–1377.

BONOTTO, S., JANOWSKI, M., VANDEN DRIESSCHE, T. and BRACHET, J. (1968) Effet spécifique de la rifampicine sur la synthèse du RNA chez *Acetabularia mediterranea*. *Arch. Intern. Physiol. Bioch.* **76**, 919–920.

BONOTTO, S. and PUISEUX-DAO, S. (1970) Modificationd e la morphologie des verticilles et différenciation chez l'*Acetabularia mediterranea*. *C. R. Acad. Sci. Paris* **270**, 1100–1104.

BOUCK, G. B. (1964) Fine structure in *Acetabularia* and its relationship to protoplasmic streaming. In *Primitive motile systems in Cell Biology*. Edrs. Allen R. D. and Kamiya, N. Academic Press, New York and London.

BRACHET, J. (1941) La localisation des acides pentosenucléiques dans les tissus animaux et les oeufs d'Amphibiens en voie de développement. *Arch. Biol.* **53**, 207–257

BRACHET, J. (1951) Quelques effets cytologiques et cytochimiques des inhibiteurs des phosphorylations oxydatives. *Experientia* **7**, 344–345.

BRACHET, J. (1952) Quelques effets des inhibiteurs des phosphorylations oxydatives sur les fragments nucléés et anucléés d'organismes unicellulaires. *Experientia* **8**, 347–351.

BRACHET, J. (1957) *Biochemical Cytology*. Academic Press, New York and London.

BRACHET, J. (1958a) The effects of Various Metabolites and Antimetabolites on the Regeneration of Fragments of *Acetabularia mediterranea*. *Exptl. Cell Res.* **12**, 639–648.

BRACHET, J. (1958b) New Observations on Biochemical Interactions

REFERENCES 143

Between Nucleus and Cytoplasm in *Amoeba* and *Acetabularia*. *Exptl. Cell Res.*, *Suppl.* 6, 78–96.

BRACHET, J. (1961) Nucleocytoplasmic Interactions in Unicellular Organisms. In *The Cell*, Edrs. Brachet, J. and Mirsky, A. E. Academic Press, New York and London.

BRACHET, J. (1962a) Effects of β-Mercaptoethanol and Lipoic Acid on Morphogenesis. *Nature* 193, 87–88.

BRACHET, J. (1962b) Nucleic Acids in Development. *J. Cell Comp. Physiol.*, *Suppl.*1 60, 1–18.

BRACHET, J. (1963a) The Role of the Nucleic Acids in the Process of Induction, Regulation and Differentiation in the Amphibian Embryo and the unicellular Alga *Acetabularia mediterranea*. In *Symposium on Biological Organization, Varenna, 1962*. Ed. Harris, R. J. C. Academic Press, New York and London, 167–182

BRACHET, J. (1963b) The Effects of Puromycin on Morphogenesis in Amphibian Eggs and *Acetabularia mediterranea*. *Nature* 199, 714–715.

BRACHET, J. (1963c) Acides ribonucléiques "messagers" et morphogenèse. *Bull. Acad. Roy. Belg.* 49, 862–887.

BRACHET, J. (1965a) Le rôle des acides nucléiques dans la morphogenèse. *L'Année Biol.* 4, 2–48.

BRACHET, J. (1965b) The Role of Nucleic Acids in Morphogenesis. *Progr. Biophys. and Molec. Biol.* 15, 99–127.

BRACHET, J. (1965c) Le contrôle de la synthèse des protéines en l'absence du noyau cellulaire. Faits et hypothèses. *Bull. Acad. Roy. Belg.* 51, 257–276.

BRACHET, J. (1967a) Protein Synthesis in the Absence of the Nucleus. *Nature* 213, 650–655.

BRACHET, J. (1967b) Effects of Hydroxyurea on Development and Regeneration. *Nature* 214, 1132–1133.

BRACHET, J. (1967c) Morphogenèse et synthèse des protéines en l'absence du noyau cellulaire. In *De l'Embryologie expérimentale à la Biologie moléculaire*. Ed. Wolff E. Dunod, Paris, 5–42.

BRACHET, J. (1968a) Quelques aspects moléculaires de la cytologie et de l'embryologie. *Biol. Reviews* 43, 1–16.

BRACHET, J. (1968b) Synthesis of Macromolecules and Morphogenesis in *Acetabularia*. In *Current Topics in Developmental Biology*, Edrs. Monroy, A. and Moscona, A. Academic Press, New York and London, 1–36.

BRACHET, J. and BRYGIER, J. (1953) Le rôle de la lumière dans la régénération et l'incorporation de CO_2 radioactif chez *Acetabularia mediterranea*. *Arch. Intern. Physiol.* 61, 246–248.

BRACHET, J. and CHANTRENNE, H. (1952) Incorporation de $^{14}CO_2$ dans les protéines des chloroplastes et des microsomes de fragments nucléés et anucléés d'*Acetabularia mediterranea*. *Arch. Intern. Physiol.* 60, 547–549.

BRACHET, J., CHANTRENNE, H. and VANDERHAEGHE, F. (1955) Recherches sur les interactions biochimiques entre le noyau et le cytoplasme chez les organismes unicellulaires. II. *Acetabularia mediterranea*. *Bioch. Bioph. Acta* 18, 544–563.

BRACHET, J., DENIS, H. and VITRY, F. de (1964) The Effects of Actinomycin D and Puromycin on Morphogenesis in Amphibian Eggs and *Acetabularia mediterranea*. *Developmental Biol.* 9, 398–434.

BRACHET, J. and GOFFEAU, A. (1964) Le rôle des acides désoxyribonucléiques (DNA) dans la synthèse des protéines chloroplastiques chez *Acetabularia mediterranea*. *C.R. Acad. Sci. Paris* 259, 2899–2909.

BRACHET, J. and LIEVENS, A. (1970) Biokhimiya (in press).

BRACHET, J. and OLSZEWSKA, M. J. (1960) Influence of localized Ultra-Violet Irradiation on the Incorporation of Adenine-8-^{14}C and DL Methionine-^{35}S in *Acetabularia mediterranea*. *Nature* 187, 954–955.

BRACHET, J. and SIX, N. (1966) Quelques observations nouvelles sur les relations entre la synthèse des acides ribonucléiques et la morphogenèse chez *Acetabularia*. *Planta* 68, 225–239.

BRACHET, J. and SZAFARZ, D. (1953) L'incorporation d'acide orotique radioactif dans les fragments nucléés et anucléés d'*Acetabularia mediterranea*. *Bioch. Bioph. Acta* 12, 588–589.

BREMER, H. J. and SCHWEIGER, H. G. (1960) Der NH_3-Gehalt kernhaltiger und kernloser Acetabularien. *Planta* 55, 13–21.

BREMER, H. J., SCHWEIGER, H. G. and SCHWEIGER, E. (1962) Das Verhaltender freien Aminosäuren in kernhaltigen und kernlosen Acetabularien. *Bioch. Bioph. Acta* 56, 380–382.

CASPERSON, T. (1941) Studien über den Eiweissumsatz der Zelle. *Naturwissenschaften* 29, 33–43.

CHANTRENNE- H., BRACHET, J. and BRYGIER, J. (1953) Quelques données nouvelles sur le rôle du noyau cellulaire dans le métabolisme des protéines chez *Acetabularia mediterranea*. *Arch. Intern. Physiol.* 61, 419–420.

CHANTRENNE, H., VAN HALTEREN, M. and BRACHET, J. (1952) La respiration de fragments nucléés et énucléés d'*Acetabularia mediterranea*. *Arch. Intern. Physiol.* 60, 187.

CLAUSS, H. (1958) Ueber quantitative Veränderungen der Chloroplasten und Cytoplasmatischen Proteine in kernlosen Teilen von *Acetabularia mediterranea*. *Planta* 52, 334–339.

CLAUSS, H. (1959) Das Verhalten der Phosphorylase in kernhaltigen und kernlosen Teilen von *Acetabularia mediterranea*. *Planta*, 52, 534–542.

CLAUSS, H. (1961) Ueber den Einbau von ^{35}S in *Acetabularia mediterranea*. *Z. Naturforsch.* 16b, 770–771.

CLAUSS, H. (1962a) Zur Frage der Beteiligung intrazellulärer Hemmfaktoren bei der Proteinsynthese von *Acetabularia*. *Z. Naturforsch.* 17b, 339–341.

CLAUSS, H. (1962b) Ueber die Intensität der Proteinsynthese von *Acetabularia* vor und nach der Hutbildung. *Z. Naturforsch.* 17b, 342–344.

CLAUSS, H. (1963) Ueber den Einfluss von Rot- und Blaulicht auf das Wachstum kernhaltiger Teile von *Acetabularia mediterranea*. *Z. Naturforsch.* 50, 719.

CLAUSS, H. (1968) Beeinflussung der Morphogenese, Substanzproduktion und Proteinzunahme von *Acetabularia mediterranea* durch sichtbare Strahlung. *Protoplasma*, 65, 49–80.

CLAUS, H. (1970) Effects of Red and Blue light on Morphogenesis and Metabolism of *Acetabularia mediterranea*. In *Biology of Acetabularia*. Edrs. Brachet, J. and Bonotto, S., Academic Press, New York and London, 177–194.

CLAUSS, H. and KECK, K. (1959) Ueber die löslichen Kohlenhydrate der Grünalge *Acetabularia mediterranea* und deren quantitative Veränderungen in kernhaltigen und kernlosen Teilen. *Planta* **52**, 543–553.

CLAUSS, H. and WERZ, G. (1961) Ueber die Geschwindigkeit der Proteinsynthese in kernlosen und kernhaltigen Zellen von *Acetabularia*. *Z. Naturforsch.* **16b**, 161–165.

CRAWLEY, J. C. (1963) The fine structure of *Acetabularia mediterranea*. *Exptl. Cell Res.* **32**, 368–378.

CRAWLEY, J. C. (1964) Cytoplasmic fine structure in *Acetabularia*. *Exptl. Cell Res.* **35**, 497–506.

CRAWLEY, J. C. (1966) Some observations on the fine structure of the gametes and zygotes of *Acetabularia*. *Planta* **69**, 365–376.

CRAWLEY, J. C. (1970) The fine structure of the gametes and zygotes of *Acetabularia*. In *Biology of Acetabularia*. Edrs. Brachet, J. and Bonotto, S. Academic Press, New York and London, 73–86.

DAO, S. (1954a) Comportement de l'*Acetabularia mediterranea* Lam. en culture. Etude de sa croissance. *Rev. Gén. Bot.* **61**, 573–606.

DAO, S. (1954b) Action de l'acide indol-acétique sur l'*Acetabularia mediterranea* Lam. en culture. *C.R. Acad. Sci., Paris* **338**, 2340–2341.

DAO, S. (1956) A propos de l'action du tryptophane sur l'*Acetabularia mediterranea* Lamour., *C.R. Acad. Sci., Paris* **243**, 1552–1554.

DAZY, A. C. (1970) Action du bromure d'éthidium sur la morphogenèse d'*Acetabularia mediterranea* et la structure de ses plastes (in preparation).

DILLARD, W. L. (1970) RNA synthesis in *Acetabularia*. In *Biology of Acetabularia*. Edrs. Brachet, J. and Bonotto, S. Academic Press, New York and London, 13–15.

DILLARD, W. L. and SCHWEIGER, H. G. (1968) Kinetics of RNA synthesis in *Acetabularia*. *Bioch. Bioph. Acta* **169**, 561–563.

DILLARD, W. L. and SCHWEIGER, H. G. (1969) RNA synthesis in *Acetabularia*. III. The kinetics of RNA synthesis in nucleate and enucleated cells. *Protoplasma* **67**, 87–100.

ERRERA, M. and VANDERHAEGHE, F. (1957) Effets des rayons UV sur *Acetabularia mediterranea*. *Exptl. Cell Res.* **13**, 1–10.

FARBER, F. E. (1969a) Studies on RNA metabolism in *Acetabularia mediterranea*. I. The isolation of RNA and labelling studies on RNA of whole plants and plant fragments. *Bioch. Bioph. Acta* **174**, 1–11.

FARBER, F. E. (1969b) *op. cit.* II. The localization and stability of RNA species; the effects on RNA metabolism of dark period and actinomycin D. *Bioch. Bioph. Acta* **174**, 12–22.

FARBER, F. E., CAPE, M., DECROLY, M. and BRACHET, J. (1968) The *in vitro* translation of *Acetabularia mediterranea* RNA. *Proc. Natl. Acad. Sci.* **61**, 843–846.

FREI, E. and PRESTON, R. D. (1968) Non-cellulosic structural polysaccharides in alga cell walls. III. Mannan in siphonous green algae. *Proc. Roy. Soc. B.* **169**, 127–145.

GIARDINA, G. (1954) Role of the Nucleus in the Maintenance of the Protein Level in the Alga *Acetabularia mediterranea. Experientia* **10**, 215.

GIBOR, A. and IZAWA, M. (1963) The DNA Content of the Chloroplasts of *Acetabularia. Proc. Nat. Acad. Sci.* **50**, 1164–1169.

GOFFEAU, A. and BRACHET, J. (1965) Deoxyribonucleic Acid-dependent Incorporation of Amino-acids in the Proteins of the Chloroplasts isolated from anucleate *Acetabularia* Fragments. *Bioch. Bioph. Acta* **95**, 302–313.

GREEN, B., BURTON, H., HEILPORN, V. and LIMBOSCH, S. (1970) The cytoplasmic DNAs of *Acetabularia*: their structure and biochemical properties. In *Biology of Acetabularia.* Edrs. Brachet, J. and Bonotto, S. Academic Press, New York and London, 35–60.

GREEN, B., HEILPORN, V., LIMBOSCH, S., BOLOUKHÈRE, M. and BRACHET, J. (1967) The cytoplasmic DNAs of *Acetabularia mediterranea. Proc. Nat. Acad. Sci.* **58**, 1351–1358.

HÄMMERLING, J. (1931) Entwicklung und Formbildungsvermögen von *Acetabularia mediterranea. Biol. Zbl.* **51**, 633–647.

HÄMMERLING, J. (1932) Entwicklung und Formbildungsvermögen von *Acetabularia mediterranea* II. Das Formbildungsvermögen kernhaltigen und kernlosen Teilstücke. *Biol. Zbl.* **52**, 42–61.

HÄMMERLING, J. (1934a) Regenerationsversuche an kernhaltigen und kernlosen Zellteilen von *Acetabularia Wettsteinii. Biol. Zbl.* **54**, 650–665.

HÄMMERLING, J. (1934b) Entwicklungsphysiologische und genetische Grundlagen der Formbildung bei der Schirmalge *Acetabularia. Naturwissenschaften* **22**, 829–836.

HÄMMERLING, J. (1934c) Ueber formbildende Substanzen bei *Acetabularia mediterranea*, ihre räumliche und zeitliche Verteilung und ihre Herkunft. *Arch. Entwicklungsmechan.* **131**, 1–81.

HÄMMERLING, J. (1934d) Ueber die Geschlechtsverhältnisse von *Acetabularia mediterranea* und *Acetabularia Wettsteinii. Arch. Protistenk.* **83**, 57–97.

HÄMMERLING, J. (1935) Ueber Genomwirkungen und Formbildungsfähigkeit bei *Acetabularia. Arch. Entwicklungsmechan.* **132**, 424–462.

HÄMMERLING, J. (1936) Studien zum Polaritätsproblem. *Zool. Jahrb.* **56**, 441–483.

HÄMMERLING, J. (1939) Ueber die Bedingungen der Kernteilung und der Zystenbildung bei *Acetabularia mediterranea. Biol. Zbl.* **59**, 158–193.

HÄMMERLING, J. (1940) Transplantationsversuche zwischen *Acetabularia mediterranea* und *Acetabularia crenulata. Note Ist. Biol. mar. Rovigno* **2**, 1.

HÄMMERLING, J. (1943a) Entwicklung und Regeneration von *Acetabularia crenulata. Zeit. Abstamm. u. Vererbungslehre* **81**, 84–113.

HÄMMERLING, J. (1943b) Ein- und zweikernige Transplantate zwischen *Acetabularia mediterranea* und *Acetabularia crenulata. Zeit. Abstamm. u. Vererbungslehre* **81**, 114–180.

HÄMMERLING, J. (1944) Zur Lebenweise, Fortpflanzung und Entwicklung verschiedener Dasycladaceae. *Arch. Protistenk.* **97**, 7–56.

HÄMMERLING, J. (1946a) Neue Untersuchungen über die physiologischen und genetischen Grundlagen der Formbildung. *Naturwissenschaften* **11**, 361–365.

HÄMMERLING, J. (1946b) Dreikernige Transplantate zwischen *Acetabularia crenulata* und *mediterranea. Z. Naturforsch.* **1**, 337–342.

HÄMMERLING, J. (1953) Nucleocytoplasmic relationships in the development of *Acetabularia. Intern. Rev. Cytol.* **2**, 475–498.

HÄMMERLING, J. (1955a) Ueber mehrkernige Acetabularien und ihre Entstehung. *Biol. Zbl.* **74**, 420–427.

HÄMMERLING, J. (1955b) Neuere Versuche über Polarität und Differenzierung bei *Acetabularia. Biol. Zbl.* **74**, 545–554.

HÄMMERLING, J. (1956) Wirkungen von UV- und Röntgenstrahlen auf kernlose und kernhaltige Teile von *Acetabularia. Z. Naturforsch.* **11b**, 217–221.

HÄMMERLING, J. (1957) Nucleus and Cytoplasm in *Acetabularia. 8e Cong. Intern. Bot., Paris, Comm. Sect.* **10**, 87–103.

HÄMMERLING, J. (1958) Ueber die wechselseitige Abhängigkeit von Zelle und Kern. *Z. Naturforsch.* **13b**, 440–448.

HÄMMERLING, J. (1963a) Nucleocytoplasmic Interactions in *Acetabularia* and other Cells. *Ann. Rev. Plant Physiol.* **14**, 65–92.

HÄMMERLING, J. (1963b) The Role of the Nucleus in Differentiation in *Acetabularia. Symposia Soc. Exptl. Biol.* **17**, 127–137.

HÄMMERLING, J., CLAUSS, H., KECK, K., RICHTER, G. and WERZ, G. (1958) Growth and Protein Synthesis in nucleated and anucleated Cells. *Exptl. Cell Res., Suppl.* **6**, 210–226.

HÄMMERLING, J. and Ch. (1959) Kernaktivität bei aufgehobener Photosynthese. *Planta* **52**, 516–527.

HÄMMERLING, J. and STICH, H. (1954) Ueber die Aufnahme von ^{32}P in kernhaltige und kernlose Acetabularien. *Z. Naturforsch.* **9b**, 149–155.

HÄMMERLING, J. and STICH, H. (1956a) Einbau und Ausbau von ^{32}P im Nukleolus (nebst Bemerkungen über intra- und extra-nukleare Proteinsynthese). *Z. Naturforsch.* **11b**, 158–161.

HÄMMERLING, J. and STICH, H. (1956b) Abhängigkeit des ^{32}P Einbaues in den Nukleolus von Energiezustand des Cytoplasmas, sowie voräufige Versuche über Kernwirkungen während der Abbauphase des Kernes. *Z. Naturforsch.* **11b**, 162–165.

HÄMMERLING, J. and WERZ, G. (1958) Ueber den Wuchsmodus von *Acetabularia. Z. Naturforsch.* **13b**, 449–454.

HEILPORN-POHL, V. and BRACHET, J. (1966) Net DNA Synthesis in anucleate fragments of *Acetabularia mediterranea. Bioch. Bioph. Acta* **119**, 429–431.

HEILPORN-POHL, V. and LIMBOSH, S. (1970) Effects of Hydroxyurea and Ethidium Bromide on *Acetabularia.* In *Biology of Acetabularia.* Edrs. Brachet, J. and Bonotto, S. Academic Press, New York and London, 61–72.

HELLEBUST, J. A., TERBORGH, J. and McLEOD, G. C. (1967) The Photosynthetic Rhythm of *Acetabularia crenulata*. II. Measurements of Photoassimilation of Carbon Dioxyd and the Activities of Enzymes of the reductive Pentose Cycle. *The Biol. Bull.* **133**, 670–678.

HOWE, M. A. (1901) Observations on the algal genera *Acicularia* and *Acetabulum. Bull. Torrey Bot. Club.* **28**, 321–334.

IRIKI, Y. and MIWA, T. (1960) Chemical Nature of the Cell Wall of the green Algae, *Codium, Acetabularia* and *Halicoryne. Nature* **185**, 178.

JANOWSKI, M. (1963) Incorporation de phosphore radioactif dans les acides ribonucléiques de fragments nucléés et anucléés d'*Acetabularia mediterranea. Arch. Intern. Physiol. Bioch.* **71**, 819–820.

JANOWSKI, M. (1965) Synthèse chloroplastique d'acides nucléiques chez *Acetabularia mediterranea. Bioch. Bioph. Acta* **103**, 399–408.

JANOWSKI, M. (1966) Detection of Ribosomes and Polysomes in *Acetabularia mediterranea. Life Sciences* **5**, 2113–2116.

JANOWSKI, M. (1967) Incorporation d'uridine-^{3}H dans les ribosomes et dans les polyribosomes d'*Acetabularia mediterranea. Arch. Intern. Physiol. Bioch.* **75**, 172.

JANOWSKI, M. and BONOTTO, S. (1970) A stable RNA species in *Acetabularia mediterranea.* In *Biology of Acetabularia.* Edrs. Brachet, J. and Bonotto, S. Academic Press, New York and London, 17–34.

JANOWSKI, M., BONOTTO, S. and BOLOUKHÈRE, M. (1969) Ribosomes of *Acetabularia. Bioch. Bioph. Acta* **174**, 525–535.

JANOWSKI, M., BONOTTO, S. and BRACHET, J. (1968) Cinétique de l'incorporation d'uridine-^{3}H dans les RNAs d'*Acetabularia mediterranea. Arch. Intern. Physiol. Bioch.* **76**, 934–935.

KECK, K. (1964) Culturing and Experimental Manipulation of *Acetabularia.* In *Methods in Cell Physiology,* Ed. Prescott, D. M. Academic Press, New York and London, **1**.

KECK, K. and CHOULES, E. A. (1963) An analysis of cellular and subcellular systems which transform the species character of acid phosphatase in *Acetabularia. J. Cell Biol.* **18**, 459–469.

KECK, K. and CLAUSS, H. (1958) Nuclear Control of Enzyme Synthesis in *Acetabularia. Bot. Gaz.* **120**, 43–49.

KLITZING, L. von (1969) Oszillatorische Regulationserscheinungen in der einzelligen Grünalge *Acetabularia. Protoplasma* **68**, 341–350.

KLITZING, L. von and SCHWEIGER, H. G. (1969) A method for Recording the circadian Rhythm of the Oxygen Balance in a Single Cell of *Acetabularia mediterranea. Protoplasma* **67**, 327–332.

LATEUR, L. (1963) Une technique de culture pour l'*Acetabularia mediterranea. Rev. Algol.* **1**, 26-37.

LEITBEG, H. (1888) Die Inkrustation der Membran von *Acetabularia. Sitzber. Akad. Wiss, Wien* **96**, 13–37.

MACKIE, W. and PRESTON, R. D. (1967) The Occurence of Mannan Microfibrils in the green Algae *Codium fragile* and *Acetabularia crenulata. Planta* **79**, 249–253.

MASCHLANKA, H. (1943) Zweikernige Transplantate zwischen *Acetabularia crenulata* und *Acicularia Schenckii. Naturwissenschaften* **31**, 549.

MASCHLANKA, H. (1946) Kernwirkung in artgleichen und artverschiedenen *Acetabularia* Transplantaten. *Biol. Zbl.* **65**, 167.

MERAC, M. L. du (1953) A propos de l'inuline des Acétabulaires. *Rev. Gén. Bot.* **60**, 689–706.

MIWA, T. (1960) Mannan and Xylan as essential Cell Wall Constituents of some siphonous green Algae. Chimie et Physico-chimie des principes immédiats tirés des Algues. *Coll. Intern., C.N.R.S. éd.*, Paris.

NAORA, H., NAORA, H. and BRACHET, J. (1960) Studies on Independent Synthesis of Cytoplasmic Ribonucleic Acids in *Acetabularia mediterranea. J. Gen. Physiol.* **43**, 1083–1102.

NAORA, H., RICHTER, G. and NAORA, H. (1959) Further studies on the synthesis of RNA in enucleate *Acetabularia mediterranea. Exptl. Cell Res.* **16**, 434–436.

NIZAMUDDIN, M. (1964) The Life History of *Acetabularia möbii* Solms-Laubach. *Annals Bot.* **28**, 77–81.

OLSZEWSKA, M. J. and BRACHET, J. (1960) Incorporation de la DL-méthionine-^{35}S dans l'Algue *Acetabularia mediterranea. Arch. Intern. Physiol. Bioch.* **68**, 693–694.

OLSZWESKA, M. J. and BRACHET, J. (1961) Incorporation de la DL-méthionine-^{35}S dans les fragments nucléés et anucléés d'*Acetabularia mediterranea. Exptl. Cell Res.* **22**, 370–380.

OLSZWESKA, M., VITRY, F. de and BRACHET, J. (1961) Influence d'irradiations UV localisées sur l'incorporation de l'adénine-8-^{14}C, de l'uridine-^{3}H et de la DL-méthionine-^{35}S dans l'Algue *Acetabularia mediterranea. Exptl. Cell Res.* **24**, 58-63.

PROVASOLI, L., McLAUGHIN, J. J. A. and DROOP, M. R. (1957) The Development of Artificial Media for marine Algae. *Arch. Mikrobiol.* **25**, 392–428.

PUISEUX-DAO, S. (1958a) Action de la ribonucléase sur le noyau de *Batophora Oerstedii* J. Ag. (Dasycladacées). *C.R. Acad. Sci. Paris* **246**, 1076–1079.

PUISEUX-DAO, S. (1958b) A propos du comportement du noyau chez le *Batophora Oerstedii* J. Ag. (Dasycladacées) cultivé, soit à l'obscurité, soit en présence de ribonucléase. *C.R. Acad. Sci. Paris* **246**, 2286–2288.

PUISEUX-DAO, S. (1960) Le comportement du noyau chez le *Batophora Oerstedii* J. Ag. (Dasycladacées) privé de lumière; ce que l'on peut en déduire sur la structure des nucléoles. *C.R. Acad, Sci. Paris* **250**, 176–178.

PUISEUX-DAO, S. (1962) Recherches biologiques et physiologiques sur quelques Dasycladacées. *Rev. Gén. Bot.* **819**, 409–503.

PUISEUX-DAO, S. (1963) Les Acétabulaires, matériel de laboratoire. *L'Année Biol. II*, **3–4**, 99–154.

PUISEUX-DAO, S. (1964) Action de la ribonucléase sur des cellules vivantes de *Mougeotia* sp. (Conjugatophycées, Chlorophycées). *J. Microsc.* **3**, 207–224.

PUISEUX-DAO, S. (1965) Morphologie et Morphogenèse chez les Dasycladacées. *Travaux dédiés à L. Plantefol.* Masson, Paris.

PUISEUX-DAO, S. (1966) L'ultrastructure et la division des plastes chez l'*Acetabularia mediterranea*, Dasycladacées. *Sixth Intern. Cong. Electron Microsc. Kyoto*, 377–378.

PUISEUX-DAO, S. (1967) The Nucleus of the Siphonales and the Siphonocladales. In *The Chromosomes of the Algae*. Ed. Godward, M. B. E. Edward Arnold, London.

PUISEUX-DAO, S. (1968) Evolution de la population des plastes chez l'*Acetabularia mediterranea*, Dasycladacées. *C.R. Acad. Sci.* **266**, 1382–1384.

PUISEUX-DAO, S. (1970) Le problème de contrôle nucléairé du fonctionnement des plastes chez l'*Acetabularia*. *C.R. Acad. Sci. Paris* **270**, 358–361.

PUISEUX-DAO, S. and DAZY, A. C. (1970) Plastid structure and the evolution of plastids in *Acetabularia*. In *Biology of Acetabularia*. Edrs. Brachet, J. and Bonotto, S., Academic Press, New York and London, 111–124.

PUISEUX-DAO, S., GIBELLO, D. and HOURSIANGOU-NEUBRUN, D. (1967) Techniques de mise en évidence du DNA dans les plastes. *C.R. Acad. Sci. Paris* **265**, 406–408.

PUISEUX-DAO, S. and GILBERT, A. M. (1967) Rythme de réplication de l'unité plastidale chez l'*Acetabularia mediterranea* placée dans diverses conditions d'éclairement. *C.R. Acad. Sci. Paris* **265**, 870–873.

PUISEUX-DAO, S. and LEVAIN, N. (1966) Morphologie ultrastructurale d'*Euglena gracilis*, cultivé en présence d'antimétabolites des substances biologiques soufrées. *Sixth Intern. Cong. Electron, Kyoto* 357–358.

REUTER, W. and SCHWEIGER, H. G. (1969) Kernkontrollierte Lactatdeshydrogenase in *Acetabularia*. *Protoplasma* **68**, 357–368.

RICHTER, G. (1957) Zur Frage der RNS-Synthese in kernlosen Teilen von *Acetabularia*. *Naturwissenschaften* **44**, 520–521.

RICHTER, G. (1958a) Das Verhalten der Plastidenpigmente in kernlosen Zellen und Teilstücken von *Acetabularia mediterranea*. *Planta* **52**, 259–275.

RICHTER, G. (1958b) Regeneration und RNS-Synthese bei der Einwirkung eines artfremden Zellkernes auf gealterte kernlose Zellteile von *Acetabularia mediterranea*. *Naturwissenschaften* **45**, 629–630.

RICHTER, G. (1959a) Die Auswirkungen der Zellkern Entfernung auf die Synthese von Ribonucleinsaüre und Cytoplasma Proteinen bei *Acetabularia mediterranea*. *Bioch. Bioph. Acta* **34**, 407–419.

RICHTER, G. (1959b) Die Auslösung kerninduzierter Regeneration bei gealterten kernlosen Zellteilen von *Acetabularia* und ihre Auswirkungen auf die Synthese von Ribonucleinsäure und Cytoplasmaproteinen. *Planta* **52**, 554–564.

RICHTER, G. (1962) Die Wirkung von blauer und roter Strahlung auf die Morphogenese von *Acetabularia*. *Naturwissenschaften* **49**, 238.

RICHTER, G. (1963) Die Tagesperiodik der Photosynthese bei *Acetabularia* und ihre Abhängigkeit von Kernaktivität, RNS- und Proteinsynthese. *Z. Naturforsch.* **18**, 1085–1089.

RICHTER, G. (1966a) Regeneration und Photosynthese-leistung kernhaltiger Zell-Teilstücke von *Acetabularia* in blauer und roter Strahlung. *Z. Pflanzenphysiol.* **54**, 106–117.

RICHTER, G. (1966b) Pulse-labelling of Nucleic Acids and Polyphosphates in Normal and Anucleate Cells of *Acetabularia*. *Nature* **212**, 1363.

SCHAEL, U. and CLAUSS, H. (1968) Die Wirkung von Rotlicht und Blaulicht auf die Photosynthese von *Acetabularia mediterranea*. *Planta* **78**, 98–114.

SCHERBAUM, O. H. (1963) Acid-soluble Phosphates in nucleate and enucleate *Acetabularia*. I. Paper-Chromatographic Patterns. *Bioch. Bioph. Acta* **72**, 509–515.

SCHERRER, K., MARCAUD, L., ZAJDELA, F., BRECKENRIDGE, B. and GROS, F. (1966) Etude des RNA nucléaires et cytoplasmiques à marquage rapide dans les cellules érythropoiétiques aviaires différenciées. *Bull. Soc. Chim. Biol.* **48**, 1037–1075.

SCHULZE, K. L. (1959) Cytologische Untersuchungen an *Acetabularia mediterranea* und *Acetabularia Wettsteinii*. *Arch. Protistenk.* **92**, 179–225.

SCHWEIGER, H. G. (1966) Ribonuclease-Aktivität in *Acetabularia*. *Planta* **68**, 247.

SCHWEIGER, H. G. (1969) Cell Biology of *Acetabularia*. In *Current Topics in Microbiology and Immunology*. Springer-Verlag, Berlin, Heidelberg and New York.

SCHWEIGER, H. G. and BERGER, S. (1964) DNA- dependent RNA Synthesis in Chloroplasts of *Acetabularia*. *Bioch. Bioph. Acta* **77**, 533–535.

SCHWEIGER, H. G. and BREMER, H. J. (1960a) Das Verhalten verschiedener P-Fraktionen in kernhaltigen und kernlosen *Acetabularia mediterranea*. *Z. Naturforsch.* **15b**, 395–400.

SCHWEIGER, H. G. and BREMER, H. J. (1960b) Nachweis cytoplasmatischer Ribonucleinsäuresynthese in kernlosen Acetabularien. *Exptl. Cell Res.* **20**, 617–618.

SCHWEIGER, H. G. and BREMER, H. J. (1961) Cytoplasmatische RNS Synthese in kernlosen Acetabularien. *Bioch. Bioph. Acta* **51**, 50–59.

SCHWEIGER, H. G., DILLARD, W. L., GIBOR, A. and BERGER, S. (1967) RNA-Synthesis in *Acetabularia*. I. RNA-Synthesis in enucleated cells. **64**, 1–12.

SCHWEIGER, H. G. and SCHWEIGER, E. (1963) Zur Wirkung von Actinomycin C auf *Acetabularia*. *Naturwissenschaften* **50**, 620–621.

SCHWEIGER, H. G., WERZ, G. and REUTER, W. (1969) Tochter-generationen von heterologen Implantaten bei *Acetabularia*. *Protoplasma* **68**, 354–356.

SCHWEIGER, E., WALRAFF, H. G. and SCHWEIGER, H. G. (1964a) Endogenous circadian Rhythm in Cytoplasm of *Acetabularia*: Influence of the Nucleus. *Science* **146**, 658–659.

SCHWEIGER, E., WALRAFF, H. G. and SCHWEIGER, H. G. (1964b) Uber tagesperiodische Schwankungen der Sauerstoffbilanz kernhaltiger und kernloser *Acetabularia mediterranea*. *Z. Naturforsch.* **19b**, 499–505.

SHEPHARD, D. (1965a) Chloroplast Multiplication and Growth in the unicellular Alga *Acetabularia mediterranea*. *Exptl. Cell Res.* **37**, 93–110.

SHEPHARD, D. (1965b) An autoradiographic Comparison of the Effects of Enucleation and Actinomycin D on the Incorporation of Nucleic

152   ACETABULARIA AND CELL BIOLOGY

Acids and Protein Precursors by *Acetabularia mediterranea*. *Bioch. Bioph. Acta* **108**, 635–643.

SHEPHARD, D. (1969) Axenic culture of *Acetabularia* in synthetic media. In *Methods in Cell Physiology* **4**, Ed. Prescott, D. Academic Press, New York and London (in press).

SHEPHARD, D. (1970) Photosynthesis in Chloroplasts isolated from *Acetabularia mediterranea*. In *Biology of Acetabularia*. Edrs. Brachet, J. and Bonotto, S., Academic Press, New York and London, 195–212.

SHEPHARD, D., LEVIN, W. B. and BIDWELL, R. G. S. (1968) Normal Photosynthesis by isolated Chloroplasts. *Bioch. Bioph. Res. Comm.* **32**, 413–420.

SIEGESMUND, K. A., ROSEN, W. G. and GAWLIK, S. T. (1962) Effect of darkness and of streptomycin on the fine structure of *Euglena gracilis*. *Amer. J. Bot.* **49**, 137–145.

SIX, E. (1956a) Die Wirkung von Strahlen auf *Acetabularia* I. Die Wirkung von Ultravioletten Strahlen auf kernlose Teile von *Acetabularia mediterranea*. *Z. Naturforsch.* **11b**, 463–470.

SIX, E. (1956b) Die Wirkung von Strahlen auf *Acetabularia*. II. Die Wirkung Röntgenstrahlen auf kernlose Teile von *Acetabularia mediterranea*. *Z. Naturforsch.* **11b**, 598–603.

SIX, E. (1958) III. Die Wirkung von Röntgenstrahlen und Ultravioletten Strahlen auf kernhaltige Teile von *Acetabularia mediterranea*. *Z. Naturforsch.* **13b**, 6–13.

SIX, E. and PUISEUX-DAO, S. (1961) Die Wirkung von Strahlen auf Acetabularien. IV. Röntgenstrahlenwirkungen in zweikernigen Transplantaten. *Z. Naturforsch.* **16b**, 832–835.

SOLMS-LAUBACH, H. (1895) Monograph of the Acetabulariae. *Trans. Linn. Soc. London Bot.*, *II* **5**, 1-39.

SPENCER, T. (1968) Effect of Kinetin on the Phosphatase Enzymes of *Acetabularia*. *Nature* **217**, 62–64.

SPENCER, T. and HARRIS, H. (1964) Regulation of Enzyme Synthesis in an Enucleate Cell. *Bioch. J.* **91**, 282–286.

STICH, H. (1951a) Experimentelle karyologische und cytochemische Untersuchungen an *Acetabularia mediterranea*. Ein Beitrag zur Beziehung zwischen Kerngrösse und Eiweissynthese. *Z. Naturforsch.* **6b**, 319–326.

STICH, H. (1951b) Trypaflavin und Ribonucleinsaüre. Untersucht an Maüsegeweben, *Condylostoma*. sp. und *Acetabularia mediterranea*. *Naturwissenschaften* **38**, 435–436.

STICH, H. (1953) Der Nachweiss und das Verhalten von Metaphosphaten in normalen, verdunkelten und Trypaflavinbehandelten *Acetabularia*. *Z. Naturforsch.* **8b**, 36–44.

STICH, H. (1956a) Anderungen von Kern und Polyphosphaten in Abhängigkeit von dem Energiegehalt des Cytoplasmas bei *Acetabularia*. *Chromosoma* **7**, 693–707.

STICH, H. (1956b) Bau und Funktion der Nukleolen. *Experientia* **12**, 7–14.

STICH, H. (1959) Changes in Nucleoli related to Alteration in Cellular

Metabolism. In *Developmental Cytology*. Ronald Press Co., New York, 105–122.

STICH, H. and HÄMMERLING, J. (1953) Der Einbau von ³²P in die Nukleolarsubstanz des Zellkernes von *Acetabularia mediterranea*. *Z. Naturforsch.* **8b**, 329–333.

STICH, H. and KITIYAKARA, A. (1957) Self-Regulation of Protein Synthesis in *Acetabularia*. *Science* **126**, 1019–1020.

STICH, H. and PLAUT, W. (1958) The Effect of Ribonuclease on Protein Synthesis in nucleated and enucleated Fragments of *Acetabularia*. *J. Bioph. Bioch. Cytol.* **4**, 1, 119–121.

SWEENEY, B. M. and HAXO, F. T. (1961) Persistence of a photosynthetic Rhythm in enucleated *Acetabularia*. *Science* **134**, 1361–1363.

TANDLER, C. J. (1962a) Oxalic Acid and Potassium in *Acetabularia*. *Naturwissenschaften* **5**, 112–114.

TANDLER, C. J. (1962b) A Naturally Occurring Crystalline Indolyl Derivative in *Acetabularia*. *Naturwissenschaften* **9**, 213–214.

TANDLER, C. J. (1962c) Bound Indole in *Acetabularia*. *Planta* **59**, 91–107.

TERBORGH, J. W. (1965) Effects of red and blue light on the Growth and Morphogenesis of *Acetabularia crenulata*. *Nature* **40**, 1360–1363.

TERBORGH, J. W. (1966) Potentiation of photosynthetic Oxygen Evolution in red Light by small Quantities of monochromatic blue Light. *Plant Physiol.* **41**, 1401–1410.

TERBORGH, J. W. and McLEOD, G. C. (1967) The photosynthetic Rhythm of *Acetabularia crenulata*. I. Continuous Measurements of Oxygen Exchange in alternating Light-Dark Regimes and in constant Light of different Intensities. *Biol. Bull.* **133**, 659–669.

TERBORGH, J. W. and THIMANN, K. V. (1964) The Effects of Light Intensity and Photoperiod on the Growth Rate, Efficiency of Growth and Chlorophyll Content of *Acetabularia crenulata*. *Planta* **63**, 83–98.

TERBORGH, J. W. and THIMANN, K. V. (1965) The Control of Development in *Acetabularia crenulata*. *Planta* **64**, 241–253.

THILO, E., GRUNZE, H., HÄMMERLING, J. and WERZ, G. (1956) Über Isolierung und Identifizierung der polyphosphate aus *Acetabularia mediterranea*. *Z. Naturforsch.* **11b**, 266–270.

THIMANN, K. V. and BETH, K. (1959) Action of Auxins on *Acetabularia* and the effect of Enucleation. *Nature* **183**, 946–948.

TRIPLETT, E. L., STEENS-LIEVENS, A. and BALTUS, E. (1965) Rates of Synthesis of Acid Phosphatases in nucleate and enucleate *Acetabularia* Fragments. *Exptl. Cell Res.* **38**, 366–379.

VALET, G. (1967) Sur l'origine endogène des rameaux verticillés chez certaines Dasycladales. *C.R. Acad. Sci. Paris* **265**, 1175–1178.

VALET, G. (1968) Contribution à l'étude des Dasycladales. 1. Morphogenèse. *Nova Hedwigia* **16**, 22–84.

VALET, G. (1969) Contribution à l'étude des Dasycladales. 2. Cytologie et reproduction. 3. Révision systématique, distribution géographique et relations phylogénétiques. *Nova Hedwigia* **17**, 551–644.

VANDEN DRIESSCHE, T. (1966a) Circadian Rhythms in *Acetabularia*. *Exptl. Cell Res.* **42**, 18–30.

VANDEN DRIESSCHE, T. (1966b) The role of the nucleus in the Circadian Rhythms of *Acetabularia mediterranea*. *Bioch. Bioph. Acta* **126**, 456–470.

VANDEN DRIESSCHE, T. (1967a) Experiments and Hypothesis on the Role of RNA in the Circadian Rhythm of Photosynthetic Capacity in *Acetabularia mediterranea*. *Nachr. Akad. Wiss. Göttingen* **10**, 108–109.

VANDEN DRIESSCHE, T. (1967b) The Nuclear Control of the Chloroplasts' Circadian Rhythms. *Sci. Prog. Oxf.* **55**, 293–303.

VANDEN DRIESSCHE, T. (1970) Temporal Regulation in Acetabularia. In *Biology of Acetabularia*. Edrs. Brachet, J. and Bonotto, S., Academic Press, New York and London, 213–238.

VANDEN DRIESSCHE, T. and BONOTTO, S. (1967) Nature du matériel accumulé par les chloroplastes d'*Acetabularia mediterranea*. *Arch. Intern. Physiol. Bioch.* **75**, 186–187.

VANDEN DRIESSCHE, T. and BONOTTO, S. (1968a) Le rythme circadien de la teneur en inuline chloroplastique d'*Acetabularia mediterranea*. *Arch. Intern. Physiol. Bioch.* **76**, 205–206.

VANDEN DRIESSCHE, T. and BONOTTO, S. (1968b) Variations journalières de l'incorporation d'uridine dans le RNA d'*Acetabularia*. *Arch. Intern. Physiol. Bioch.* **76**, 919–920.

VANDEN DRIESSCHE, T. and BONOTTO, S. (1969) The circadian rhythm in, RNA synthesis in *Acetabularia mediterranea*. *Bioch. Bioph. Acta* **179**, 58–66.

VANDERHAEGHE, F. (1952) Mesures de croissance de fragments nucléés et anucléés d'*Acetabularia mediterranea*. *Arch. Intern. Physiol.* **60**, 190.

VANDERHAEGHE, F. (1954) Les effets de l'énucléation sur la synthèse des protéines chez *Acetabularia mediterranea*. *Bioch. Bioph. Acta* **15**, 281–287.

VANDERHAEGHE, F. (1957) Thesis, University of Brussels.

VANDERHAEGHE-HOUGARDY, F. and BALTUS, E. (1968) Effets de l'énucléation sur le maintien de la phosphatase acide dans le cytoplasme d'*Acetabularia mediterranea*. *Arch. Intern. Physiol. Bioch.* **70**, 414–415.

VANDERHAEGHE, F. and SAFARZ, D. (1955) Enucleation et synthèse d'acide ribonucléique chez *Acetabularia mediterranea*. *Arch. Intern. Physiol.* **63**, 267–268.

VAN GANSEN, P. and BOLOUKHÈRE-PRESBURG, M. (1965) Ultrastructure de l'Algue unicellulaire *Acetabularia mediterranea*. *J. Microsc.* **4**, 347–362.

VITRY, F. de (1962a) Etude de l'action de la 5-fluorodéoxyuridine sur la croissance et la morphogenèse d'*Acetabularia mediterranea*. *Exptl. Cell Res.* **25**, 697–699.

VITRY, F. de (1962b) Action des métabolites et antimétabolites sur la croissance et la morphogenèse d'*Acetabularia mediterranea*. *Protoplasma* **55**, 313–319.

VITRY, F. de (1963) Etude autoradiographique de l'incorporation de la ^{3}H-5-méthylcytosine chez *Acetabularia mediterranea*. *Exptl. Cell Res.* **31**, 376–381.

VITRY, F. de (1964a) Etude autoradiographique de l'incorporation de l'actinomycine ^{14}C chez *Acetabularia mediterranea*. *C.R. Acad. Sci., Paris* **258**, 4829–4831.

VITRY, F. de (1964b) Etude autoradiographique des effets de la 5-fluoro-déoxyuridine, de l'actinomycine et de la puromycine chez *Acetabularia mediterranea. Deve. Biol.* **9**, 484–504.

VITRY, F. de (1965a) Etude du métabolisme des acides nucléiques chez *Acetabularia mediterranea.* I. Incorporation de précurseurs de DNA, de RNA et de protéines chez *Acetabularia mediterranea. Bull. Soc. Chim. Biol.* **47**, 1325–1351.

VITRY, F. de (1965b) *Op. cit.* II. Mise en évidence du DNA nucléaire à l'aide du phényléthylalcool, de la FUDR. Effets biologiques de l'actino-mycine D et de la puromycine. *Bull. Soc. Chim. Biol.* **47**, 1352–1372.

VITRY, F. de (1965c) *Op. cit.* III. Etude autoradiographique des effets de l'actinomycine D et de la puromycine. *Bull. Soc. Chim. Biol.* **47**, 1372–1394.

WERZ, G. (1955) Kernphysiologische Untersuchungen an *Acetabularia.* I–III. *Planta* **46**, 113–153.

WERZ, G. (1957a) Membranbildung bei kernlosen wachsenden und nicht wachsenden Teilen von *Acetabularia mediterranea. Z. Naturforsch.* **12b**, 739–740.

WERZ, G. (1957b) Eiweissvermehrung in ein- und zweikernigen Systemen von *Acetabularia. Experientia* **13**, 79.

WERZ, G. (1957c) Ueber die Wirkung von Cobalt-II-nitrat auf Kern und Cytoplasma von *Acetabularia mediterranea. Experientia* **13**, 279–284.

WERZ, G. (1957d) Die Wirkung von Trypaflavin auf Kern und Cyto-plasma von *Acetabularia mediterranea. Z. Naturforsch.* **12b**, 559–563.

WERZ, G. (1959) Weitere Untersuchungen zum Problem der Kernaktivität bei gesenkten Zellstoffwechsel. *Planta* **53**, 528–532.

WERZ, G. (1960a) Anreicherung von Ribonucleinsaüre in der Wuchszone von *Acetabularia mediterranea. Planta* **55**, 22–37.

WERZ, G. (1960b) Ueber Strukturierungen der Wuchszone von *Aceta-bularia mediterranea. Planta* **55**, 38–56.

WERZ, G. (1961a) Unterschiede der Protoplasten-Strukturungen bei verschieden Dasycladaceen und ihre Abhängigkeit von artspezifischen Kernwirkungen. *Planta* **56**, 490–498.

WERZ, G. (1961b) Ueber die Beeinflussung der Formbildung von *Aceta-bularia* durch Selenat. *Planta* **57**, 250–257.

WERZ, G. (1961c) Zur Frage der Herkunft und Verteilung cytoplasmati-schen Ribonucleinsäure und ihrer Beziehungen zu 'Morphogenetischen Substanzen' bei *Acetabularia mediterranea. Z. Naturforsch.* **16b**, 126–129.

WERZ, G. (1962) Zur Frage der Elimination von Ribonucleinsäure und Protein aus den Zellkern von *Acetabularia mediterranea. Planta* **57**, 636–655.

WERZ, G. (1963a) Morphogenetische Wirkungen von Aminosäure bei Acetabularien. I. Wirkungen von 3-C-Aminosäuren und verwandten Derivaten. *Planta* **60**, 205–210.

WERZ, G. (1963b) *Op. cit.* II. Die Beeinflussung der Morphogenese durch einige 4-C-Aminosäuren. *Planta* **60**, 211–215.

WERZ, G. (1963c) Vergleichende Zellmembraneanalysen bei verschiedenen Dasycladaceen. *Planta* **60**, 322–330.

WERZ, G. (1965) Determination and Realization of Morphogenesis in *Acetabularia. Brookhaven Symposia in Biol.* **18**, 185–203.

WERZ, G. (1966a) Morphologische Veränderungen in Chloroplasten und Mitochondrien von verdunkelten *Acetabularia*-Zellen. *Planta* **68**, 256–268.

WERZ, G. (1966b) Primärvorgänge bei der Realisation der Morphogenese von *Acetabularia. Planta* **69**, 53–57.

WERZ, G. (1967) Induktion von Zellwandbildung durch Fremdprotein bei *Acetabularia. Naturwissenschaften* **14**, 374–375.

WERZ, G. (1968) Plasmatische Formbildung als Voraussetzung für die Zellwandbildung bei der Morphogenese von *Acetabularia. Protoplasma* **65**, 81–96.

WERZ, G. and HÄMMERLING, J. (1959) Proteinsynthese in wachsenden und nicht wachsenden kernlosen Zellteilen von *Acetabularia. Planta* **53**, 145–161.

WERZ, G. and HÄMMERLING, J. (1961) Ueber die Beeinflussung artspezifischer Formbildungsprozesse von *Acetabularia* durch UV-Bestrahlung. *Z. Naturforsch.* **16b**, 829–832.

WERZ, G. and KELLNER, G. (1968a) Isolierung und elektronenmikroskopische Charakterisierung von Desoxyribonucleinsäure aus Chloroplasten kernloser *Acetabularia*-Zellen. *Z. Naturforsch.* **23b**, 1018a.

WERZ, G. and KELLNER, G. (1968b) Molecular characteristics of Chloroplast DNA of *Acetabularia* cells. *J. Ultrastr. Res.* **24**, 109–115.

WERZ, G. and ZETSCHE, K. (1962) Autoradiographische Untersuchungen an verdunkelten einkernigen Transplantaten von *Acetabularia mediterranea. Planta* **59**, 563–566.

WOODCOCK, C. L. and BOGORAD, L. (1968) Evidence for wide Disparity in the Amount of DNA per Plastid in *Acetabularia mediterranea. 8th Ann. Meeting of the Am. Soc. for Cell Biol.* 144a.

WOODCOCK, C. L. and BOGORAD, L. (1969) Evidence for Variation in the Quantity of DNA among Plastids of *Acetabularia, J. Cell Biol.* **44**, 361–375.

ZETSCHE, K. (1962) Die Aktivität implantierter Zellkerne von *Acetabularia* bei aufgehobener Photosynthese. *Naturwissenschaften* **17**, 404–405.

ZETSCHE, K. (1963a) Der Einfluss von Kinetin und Giberellin auf die Morphogenese kernhaltiger und kernloser Acetabularien. *Planta* **59**, 624–634.

ZETSCHE, K. (1963b) Das morphologische und physiologische Verhalten implantierter Zellkerne bei *Acetabularia mediterranea. Planta* **60**, 331–338.

ZETSCHE, K. (1964a) Der Einfluss von Actinomycin D auf die Abgabe morphogenetischer Substanzen aus dem Zellkern von *Acetabularia mediterranea. Naturwissenschaften* **51**, 18–19.

ZETSCHE, K. (1964b) Hemmung der Synthese morphogenetischer Substanzen in Zellkern von *Acetabularia mediterranea* durch Actinomycin D. *Z. Naturforsch.* **19b**, 751–759.

ZETSCHE, K. (1965a) Anreicherung von morphogenetischen Substanzen in

Lichtpflanzen von *Acetabularia mediterranea* unter dem Einfluss von Puromycin. *Planta* **64**, 119–128.

ZETSCHE, K. (1965b) Nachweiss von Guanosindiphosphat-mannose- und Uridin-diphosphateglucose Pyrophosphorylase in *Acetabularia mediterranea*. *Planta* **64**, 129–137.

ZETSCHE, K. (1966a) Anreicherung von Proteinsynthese induzierenden Substanzen in *Acetabularia mediterranea* unter dem Einfluss von Puromycin. *Z. Naturforsch.* **21b**, 88–90.

ZETSCHE, K. (1966b) Nachweis von Enzyme des Galactosestoffwechsels in der Grünalge *Acetabularia mediterranea*. *Planta* **68**, 240–246.

ZETSCHE, K. (1966c) Entkopplung morphogenetischer Prozesse in *Acetabularia mediterranea* durch P-fluorphenylalanin. *Planta* **68**, 360–370.

ZETSCHE, K. (1966d) Regulation der zeitlichen Aufeinanderfolge von Differenzierungsvorgängen bei *Acetabularia*. *Z. Naturforsch* **21b**, 375–379.

ZETSCHE, K. (1966e) Regulation der UDP-Glucose 4-Epimerase Synthese in kernhaltigen und kernlosen Acetabularien. *Bioch. Bioph. Acta* **124**, 332–338.

ZETSCHE, K. (1967) Unterschieldliche Zuzammensetzung von Stiel- und Hutzellwand bei *Acetabularia mediterranea*. *Planta* **76**, 326–334.

ZETSCHE, K. (1968) Regulation der UDPG-Pyrophosphorylaseaktivität in *Acetabularia*. I. Morphogenese und UDPG-Pyrophosphorylase-Synthese in kernhaltigen und kernlosen Zellen. *Z. Naturforsch.* **23b**, 369–376.

ZETSCHE, K. (1969a) *op. cit.* II. Unterschiedliche Synthese des Enzymes in verschiedenen Zellregionen. *Planta* **89**, 244–253.

ZETSCHE, K. (1969b) Die Wirkung von RNA- und Proteininhibitoren auf den Chlorophyllgehalt kernhaltiger und kernloser Acetabularien. *Planta* **89**, 284–298.

Index